To Kristen
Happ[...]
Love,
Mom
2-12-05

NO WHITE AT NIGHT

NO WHITE AT NIGHT

THE THREE-RULE DIET

• • •

BILL GAVIN, M.D.

RIVERHEAD BOOKS
a member of Penguin Group (USA) Inc.
New York • 2004

Every effort has been made to ensure that the information contained in this book is complete and accurate. However, neither the publisher nor the author is engaged in rendering professional advice or services to the individual reader. The ideas, procedures, and suggestions contained in this book are not intended as a substitute for consulting a physician. All matters regarding your health require medical supervision. Neither the author nor the publisher shall be liable or responsible for any loss, injury, or damage allegedly arising from any information or suggestion in this book.

The recipes contained in this book are to be followed exactly as written. The publisher is not responsible for your specific health or allergy needs that may require medical supervision. The publisher is not responsible for any adverse reactions to the recipes contained in this book.

Riverhead Books
a member of
Penguin Group (USA) Inc.
375 Hudson Street
New York, NY 10014

First published in 2003 by Eld Inlet Publishing LLC
First Riverhead edition 2004

Published simultaneously in Canada

An application has been submitted to register
this book with the Library of Congress.

ISBN 1-57322-291-7

Printed in the United States of America
1   3   5   7   9   10   8   6   4   2
This book is printed on acid-free paper. ∞

BOOK DESIGN BY TANYA MAIBORODA

To my parents for their love and guidance
To my wife for her love and encouragement
To my children for making me look like a good father

ACKNOWLEDGMENTS

THIS BOOK IS the result of years of caring for patients and friends. First, I would like to thank all of them for their help in showing me what worked and what did not for people trying to lose weight. They also showed me the public's need for a weight-loss approach that was simple. That ultimately led to the first edition of this book. Tom and Cheryl helped me edit it and put it in the proper form. Tom and Michele proofread it and gave me new ideas. Steve produced some great photos, and the people at Gorham printing made it all work.

This version of the book could not have been possible without the work of Zita, Jacki, and Linnea. Paige Cady, R.D., gave me guidance from the start and helped provide the nutritional facts. This version of the book is a significant improvement over the first edition. The basic message of the book, though, remains unchanged. Finally, I would like to thank Amy Hertz and David Black, for helping me take this message to a new level.

CONTENTS

INTRODUCTION

YOU PROBABLY BOUGHT this book because you or a loved one is overweight. Congratulations, you have taken the first step toward managing the problem. In this book I will review the causes of obesity and outline several simple steps you can take toward overcoming your weight problem. It will not be easy, but once you understand the reasons people gain weight, you will find it is not that hard to lose weight.

There is no simple pill or injection to cure obesity. There are usually multiple causes of an individual's gaining weight, and they will all need to be addressed. You will not learn *a diet* as you read this book. You will, however, learn a healthy approach to eating and exercise. The good news is that my patients who have achieved success through this approach routinely come back and tell me, "It is not that hard."

This book in part has been a personal journey for me as well. If you were to look at me now, you would find it hard to believe that I ever had a weight problem. My current height is six feet one and my weight is 167 pounds. I weighed approximately 10 pounds less and was at least one foot shorter when I was in seventh grade. I was able to get my weight under control before I entered high school, and I did not really have a weight problem again until I was about thirty-five years old. From the age of thirty-five, I relentlessly gained 3 to 5 pounds per year. Finally, when I reached a weight of 210 pounds, I decided that was enough. It was time to lose weight.

Some of the initial approaches that I used failed. I, like many of my patients, assumed that I was overweight because I was not getting enough exercise. Although I significantly increased my workout frequency, the weight loss that I achieved was minimal.

I did change my diet at the start of this effort. My prior diet could be described as "low fat," but unfortunately it was not low in calories. I gave up red meat and even started to go for lunch to the hospital, where I would typically have rice and vegetables. I remember two things about that time: I did not lose much weight and I was always hungry.

Finally, I heard about some different approaches to diet and exercise. I listened to a physician talk about the Zone diet and I thought the principles made sense. I tried to follow the diet without getting caught up in the weighing of food or other calculations. The effects were dramatic. I had only been able to lose 10 pounds over the course of a year with my initial diet changes and increased exercise. With the new changes in my diet and the same exercise program I was able to lose 35 more pounds in a year.

As I lost weight I realized how many people were looking for some help to do the same. My friends asked me for advice. Then my mother, who has struggled with her weight for a good part of her life, asked me to help her. She had been diagnosed with diabetes and had gained significant weight on some new medications for her elevated blood sugar.

I am happy to say that my mother achieved significant success with the principles of this book. She has lost 35 pounds and is no longer taking any medications for diabetes. When her friends ask her how she did it, she pulls out a copy of my book, which she always carries in her purse. That is as good as it gets.

As I lost weight, I realized that I had significant misconceptions about the roles of diet and exercise and the roles that they played in weight loss. Initially I thought that I had an exercise problem. Then I made changes in my diet that did not achieve significant weight loss, but I thought that I was eating the "right" foods. Finally, it was a two-year commitment before I was able to achieve the results that I wanted. So, I have come to understand what it means to be overweight and how challenging it can be to face the task of losing weight.

In my professional life as a cardiologist, I have seen the

number of obese patients with various types of cardiovascular disease dramatically increase. Obesity is a major cause of hypertension, diabetes, and high cholesterol levels. All of those diseases are major causes of coronary artery disease, heart attacks, and heart failure. In my office, on any given day, I usually counsel up to 30 percent or more of my patients about weight loss and diet. Initially, I recommended various programs, such as Weight Watchers, or books, such as *The Zone Diet*.[1] What I found was both surprising and challenging.

Patients came back to my office saying they could not understand the various books they had purchased, they did not want to have to go to specific group meetings, and the multiple different types of diets and various guidelines available in the public media confused them. My patients did not understand the differences between the diets, and subsequently, they really could not then determine which one was right for them. The difficulties experienced by my patients reminded me of my own shortcomings in understanding my prior diet and exercise pattern. It occurred to me that I had a lot more training in nutrition and physiology than my patients did; therefore, if I had significant misconceptions at the start of my weight-loss program, I really should not be surprised that my patients were having difficulty as well.

I discovered two important points about my patients in this process. They wanted their weight-loss program to be simple: they did not want to have to weigh their individual food portions, they did not want to buy special foods, they did not want to make recipes from unfamiliar cookbooks, and they did not want to attend special meetings. The other point I discovered was how successful my patients could be in approaching weight loss if they understood the process. Whenever I could help my patients understand what the elements were that had caused them to gain weight, and how those elements could be individually changed, they had a significant improvement in weight-loss success. So, I distilled down the important concepts of various diet programs and began recommending the principles defined in this book. These principles worked for the majority of my patients, and I believe they will work for you, too.

First, we need to review the role of a number of factors such as exercise, genetics, and the role various food groups play in your diet. My reason for putting these chapters early in the book is to help you better understand the causes of obesity. Only after you understand the causes of obesity can you adequately address them in the long term.

As a physician, I have some misgivings about the validity of my approach. In medicine, new treatments are often subjected to large, randomized trials involving thousands of patients. In this type of study, some patients are treated and others serve as controls. It is a good approach and the fundamental basis for scientific evaluation in medicine. Unfortunately, this type of study has not been done for my diet principles or on a controlled basis between many of the popular diets that are currently available to the public. I would welcome anyone to fund such a trial.

As the problem of obesity gains more attention in the medical community, I suspect the government will ultimately fund patient treatment studies of this type. But even without a major study, I can say that my diet principles have been tested. These principles have been tested on myself with success. As I lost weight, my friends initially asked if I was okay. When I reassured them that my health was fine, they all wanted to know what I was doing to lose weight. So, after myself, these diet principles were tested on my friends, and then on my patients. I can now say I have hundreds of patients and friends who have been able to overcome their weight problems and significantly improve their health through weight loss. The success of these people and their encouragement led me to write this book. I believe this book can help you as well.

The challenge in writing this book is to transfer the experience that you would have as a patient in my office into these pages. If you visit with me in my office, I have the ability to explain concepts and, more important, answer your questions. The advantage to the book is that there is more time to explain the important concepts of obesity, exercise, and weight loss. The downside is that I cannot answer your specific questions directly. In counseling hundreds of patients over the last few years, I have come to understand the most common questions and have tried to address them in this book. When patients leave my office, they have a copy of my three rules, but I also make sure they have concrete options for all three meals that include foods they like. By the time you finish this book you should also know what you will have for breakfast, lunch, and dinner on a routine basis.

There is an old Chinese proverb that a journey of a

thousand miles starts with a single step. Your first step was to recognize that you or your loved one has a significant weight problem. Buying the book is another step. Reading this book alone will not allow you to lose weight. Reading this book and following the principles regarding diet and exercise will. As you read the book, think about when you started to gain weight or noticed that you had a weight problem. Think about what changed in your diet in the years prior to that. Start watching what you are eating, and especially start reading the labels of the foods that you are eating. Then you can begin to apply the principles of the book. You did not become overweight in a day, and it will take you a considerable amount of time to lose your weight. You can lose the weight, though, and you should enjoy the journey.

1

THE SUPERSIZING OF AMERICA

AMERICANS YOUNG AND OLD are getting fat. This medical fact has been discussed in the scientific literature for years and now is being actively covered in the popular press. I have seen major stories on the obesity problem in the *Wall Street Journal, Newsweek,* and *Prevention* magazine. The government has even changed the tax code to allow deductions for the cost of weight-loss therapies. The problem of obesity is now clearly on the radar screen of America, and I hope it will be better addressed.

In 1980, the National Center for Health Statistics considered 46 percent of U.S. adults overweight or obese. *Obesity* is defined as being 20 percent above your ideal body weight. In 1999, the same group found that number had climbed to 60 percent.[2] The problem is not limited to adults. The Centers for Disease Control (CDC) has declared obesity in children an epidemic. You really do not need to read the statistics to understand the magnitude of the problem. One need only look at the people in the supermarket or the public schools to see that a major problem exists.

The impact of obesity on your health is enormous. Obesity is a major cause of high cholesterol (hypercholesterolemia or hyperlipidemia), diabetes mellitus, and hypertension. These three illnesses are recognized risk factors for cardiovascular disease. Cardiovascular disease is the leading cause of death in the United States and most Western industrialized countries. For this reason, the surgeon general has declared that obesity now ranks only behind smoking as the health factor contributing to the greatest number of premature deaths in the United States.

The impact of obesity extends far beyond cardiovascular disease. Obese people are more likely to have arthritis, require joint replacements, or sustain disabling back injuries. Obesity prevents the early detection of problems such as breast cancer and abdominal aortic aneurysm. Both of these illnesses can have fatal consequences if not detected early. Thus, obesity can contribute to both premature death and disability. To help put it in quantifiable terms for the American public, a recent study in the *Journal of the American Medical Association* found that obese individuals had a significant reduction in life expectancy.[3] For example, the life expectancy of young white males who are obese is shortened by an average of thirteen years.

Ironically, many people do seem to understand that they have a weight problem and try to address it. Americans are preoccupied with dieting and exercise. At any given time, 44 percent of women and 29 percent of men are said to be dieting.[4] The United States leads the world in the number of health clubs. So one needs to ask why Americans are having such poor outcomes in addressing their weight-control problem.

The causes of the obesity epidemic are probably multifactorial. As we have become a more technologically oriented society, we have also become a more sedentary society. A decreased energy expenditure on a daily basis without any change in diet will lead to a slow, progressive weight gain. Decreased energy expenditure is not the only cause of obesity; otherwise, exercise programs would resolve the issue. The fact is, most Americans are eating too many calories.

Food is plentiful and inexpensive in America. The USDA and other dietary advisory groups have recommended that Americans consume low-fat foods, and these groups appear to have had significant success in getting their message to the American people. Most patients I see who are overweight do not consume high-fat foods. My patients predominantly have a sedentary lifestyle and they consume an excessive amount of high-calorie, low-fat carbohydrates. Unfortunately, many people believe that they can consume unlimited quantities of low-fat foods such as pasta and potatoes. You *can* get fat eating low-fat foods in unlimited quantities.

In summary, America has a major problem with obesity. The cause of the problem is multifactorial. Unfortunately, the solutions adopted by many Americans in their diet and exercise patterns are not successful, at least over the long term. Before we review the potential solutions through diet and exercise, we need to review some further issues as contributors to the obesity problem.

2

EVOLUTION AND GENETICS

NATURE HAS GIVEN US the ability to store calories as body fat. As noted earlier, obesity is now a major health risk. You may wonder why we need to be able to accumulate body fat. The simplest answer to the question is that nature has given us a tool for survival.

Throughout the thousands of years that humans have evolved, humankind has faced a major threat—famine. We live in a unique time and place in history. Food is plentiful in the United States, but it was not always. In 1609, more than 50 percent of the early Jamestown colonists starved to death in their second year of settlement. In many parts of the world today, famine is still a major cause of death. The UN has recognized that sixteen million people were threatened by famine in southern Africa over the last year.[5] The unique combination of floods and drought, as well as a failure by the government to adequately import maize, contributed to the worst food shortage in a decade. Worldwide, the number of people at risk for famine is considerably greater in any given year. To help us survive these times of food deprivation, it is necessary to have stored energy. In the human body, energy is predominantly stored as fat.

The ability to store fat also may have played a role in ensuring survival of the species through reproduction. Women in general have a higher percentage of body fat than men. That is important for a woman's ability to carry a pregnancy to term and to nurse a newborn. Women who are malnourished stop menstruating and therefore lose the ability to reproduce. Thus, nature has probably given us the ability to store body fat to enable us to survive famine and also help ensure propagation of the species. The biochemical processes that determine our ability to store body fat are in our genetic code.

All the biochemical reactions that occur in the body are determined by our individual genetic makeup. Half of your genes or chromosomes come from your mother and the other half from your father. I believe that the ability to store body fat is a genetic trait. Some people have a stronger ability to store fat than others. If you want to know whether you have a tendency to get fat, look at your parents. I believe my own family is an excellent example.

My mother is a heavyset woman of German/Slovak descent. My father is a thin Irishman. My mother has a very strong tendency to gain weight and has struggled with her weight over the years. My father has never had a weight problem over any significant period of time. My mother has tried various diet programs and actually achieved the most success through Weight Watchers. When I was a child, a typical story in the Gavin household was that when my mother went on a diet, my father would lose weight. Although you might think that my mother would be quite happy with my father's ability to remain thin, she actually became quite angry. When Mom was unhappy it was usually not an easy time for the men in the Gavin household. I would say that story played out at least every other year in the Gavin family.

My brothers and I are nearly a perfect example of Mendelian genetic principles. There are five boys in the Gavin family. One brother looks like my mother, one brother looks like my father, and three of the brothers are blends of our two parents. The brother who looks like my mother has a significant weight problem, and the brother who resembles my father has always tended to be thin. The three blends have a tendency to vary their weight to the two greatest extremes. I am a blend.

Just as some people seem genetically more likely to gain weight through obesity, other people never seem to gain weight. In our office we have one receptionist who is in her late twenties and is a mother. She is a true size 2. One day I sat down next to her at lunch and was amazed to see that she ate roughly twice as much as I did. Fortunately, she lives in a food-plentiful society. If she or my father had been in the Jamestown colony at the time of the famine, I doubt that either of them would have lived to see the springtime. I think my mother would have made it. Just as the United States is a very favorable place for people who do not have a very good ability to store body fat, it is a very hostile place for people who have a strong tendency to gain weight, such as my mother or brother.

Genetics are important not just for our ability to store body fat. Our genetic structure was also determined by the diet of our ancestors. DNA analysis has shown that the human genome has not changed appreciably for the last two million years. An excellent review of the diet of our ancestors is *The Paleo Diet,* by Loren Cordain.[6] The diet of our ancestors had lean protein from sources such as wild game and fish. It was low in saturated fat and high in polyunsaturated fats and omega-3 fatty acids. Their diet was also high in fiber, vitamins, and antioxidants from fruit and plants. Finally, their diet was low in sugar and did not have any significant grain products.

Grain products have been in the human food supply only for the last ten thousand years. In the last thirty years the American population has been subjected to food products with increasing amounts of sugar as well as increasing amounts of fat. The increased sugar and fat levels make the foods you eat more energy-dense. Our bodies are simply not designed for a diet that is relatively high in sugar and modified fat. When we eat these "new foods" and have excess calorie intake, those extra calories are stored as fat. These foods have contributed to the epidemic of obesity and diabetes. Thus, our genetics determine not only fat storage but also the types of foods that we should eat.

The important point in understanding how genetics affects obesity is to recognize that we are all unique individuals. Part of our individual variability is expressed in our tendency to store body fat. Simply having a predisposition to store body fat does not condemn you to being obese. It does, however, force you to be much more conscious of what you are eating and what impact the foods you consume have on your body weight. If you have a strong tendency toward obesity, that tendency will never go away. You were born with your genetic structure, and it is with you for your entire life. For that reason you have to learn what foods are *right* for you and think about learning *how* to eat for a lifetime.

3

EXERCISE

EVERYONE SHOULD HAVE an exercise program. People who exercise on a routine basis often note an improved sense of well-being. Exercise will help reduce your blood sugar and blood pressure and raise your good cholesterol level. In contrast to obesity, the positive aspects of exercise will help reduce your risk of cardiovascular disease. I have tried to maintain some type of daily exercise pattern since I was in high school, and I continue to this day. I have learned that if you are overweight, it is not likely to be from lack of exercise alone.

Overweight patients who come to see me often believe that the cause of their obesity is lack of exercise. I should point out that most of my patients are in their forties or older. Sometimes my male patients have retired from physically demanding jobs in construction or the wood products industry. If you look at the calories that can be burned through exercise in Table 1 (see below), you will note that it is hard to control your weight with exercise alone. To achieve weight loss of 30 pounds a year requires burning an extra 390 calories per day. As most of my patients are limited to walking as their predominant form of exercise, getting that target of 390 calories daily would be very difficult. There is another reason I have come to believe that exercise alone will not lead to successful long-term weight loss: I've tried it. Let me tell you my personal experience.

TABLE 1 Calories Expended for Various Activities*	
Standing	104 cal/hr
Walking—2 mph	264 cal/hr
Walking—3 mph	352 cal/hr
Walking—4.5 mph	484 cal/hr
Jogging—5.5 mph	814 cal/hr
Biking—6 mph	264 cal/hr
Biking—12 mph	451 cal/hr
Swimming—25 yd/min	302 cal/hr
Jumping rope	550 cal/hr
Stair-climbing machine	300–600 cal/hr
Elliptical trainer	300–600 cal/hr
*Based on 165-pound individual.	

When I reached 210 pounds, I assumed that I was over-weight because I was not getting enough exercise. At that time I was exercising four or five days a week, usually on a Lifecycle exercise machine. I used that machine for at least thirty minutes every day I worked out. In spite of my exercise program, I found that my weight was going up relentlessly 3 to 5 pounds per year. I resolved that I would exercise more and started exercising seven days per week. I also rotated my exercise routine between the Lifecycle exercise bike and an elliptical trainer, an exercise machine designed to mimic running but with a reduced knee and hip joint impact. The elliptical trainer has a higher calorie expenditure due to its similarity to running.

I lost 10 pounds in the next six months through that change in my exercise pattern. After that, my weight plateaued, and I maintained that weight for an additional six months. At the end of the six months of being in a steady state, I changed my diet. Over the next fourteen months I lost 35 more pounds. During the time I lost the additional weight, I kept my exercise pattern at the same higher level. But changing my diet combined with exercise gave me the most success. The bottom line is that it is nearly impossible for the average person to exercise their way out of a bad diet.

Another example of this principle is what I often overhear when working out at our local health club. I work out alone, but a number of people get counseling from personal health trainers. A comment I have heard often is, "I've been doing this for two months now and haven't lost any weight." I think these people haven't yet realized that they have to change their diet as well as their exercise pattern to lose weight.

The illustration in Table 2 (see page 15) shows the dramatic effect of combining exercise with diet. I will assume that the people in the health club frustrated with their lack of weight loss were motivated to initiate their exercise programs not only to improve their fitness but to lose weight. So let's say that they are on a diet and exercise program that led them to gain 5 pounds per year. If you change your exercise pattern to lose 10 pounds per year, this is a significant and positive step. What the person experiences, though, is a weight loss of only 5 pounds per year, as half of the weight loss of the improved exercise program is canceled by the weight gain mediated by their chronic diet pattern.

The dramatic effect of combining exercise and diet is shown in the second illustration in the table. If we take the same person who is gaining 5 pounds per year and change their diet to allow them to lose 10 pounds per year through their diet alone, they will quadruple their overall weight loss. That person now is losing 10 pounds a year through exercise and 10 pounds per year through diet. The weight loss that can be achieved through exercise is markedly amplified through changing your diet.

As I said earlier, everyone should have an exercise program. Walking by itself is a great form of exercise. A recent study published in the *Journal of the American Medical Association* looked at postmenopausal women and the impact of exercise on their weight.[7] The predominant form of exercise was walking. These women lost between 2 and 8 pounds

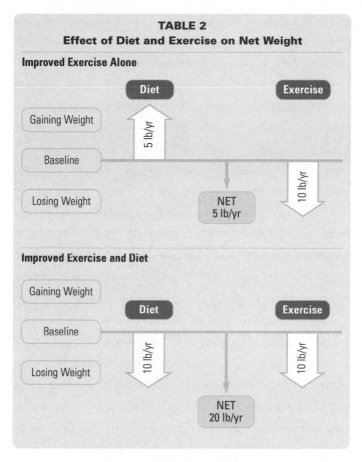

TABLE 2
Effect of Diet and Exercise on Net Weight

Improved Exercise Alone

| Diet | Exercise |

Gaining Weight

5 lb/yr

Baseline

Losing Weight

NET
5 lb/yr

10 lb/yr

Improved Exercise and Diet

Gaining Weight

| Diet | Exercise |

Baseline

Losing Weight

10 lb/yr

10 lb/yr

NET
20 lb/yr

per year. I think this is very realistic and applicable to the patients that I see in my practice all the time. For many of my arthritic or cardiac patients, walking is the only exercise they can do.

Some of my patients, unfortunately, are not even able to participate in a walking program. Typically these patients are limited due to some orthopedic problem such as significant hip or knee disease. For those patients, I recommend a television show titled *Sit and Be Fit,* which is specifically designed for them. In our local community it is provided through PBS. If you are interested, ask your local cable or satellite provider about its availability. Videotapes of the show are also available and can be obtained over the Internet. Even if you are unable to walk, there are still fitness programs available to you.

Recently the Institute of Medicine recommended that people get moderate physical activity for sixty minutes per day. This recommendation does not necessarily mean one hour of constant exercise. It can incorporate intermittent bursts of walking or stair climbing at work to total sixty minutes during the entire day. Since 1996, the surgeon general has recommended thirty minutes of exercise per day.

I recommend to my patients that they walk at least thirty minutes per day. Whatever type of exercise you choose, make sure that it works for your individual schedule. I work out in the early morning because that is a predictable part of my day when I am unlikely to be called away to take care of patients. If you can get to an exercise facility, great, but if you cannot, try walking at work. Park ten minutes away from your workplace if safety allows it, and then you will walk twenty minutes every day to and from work. Or take a walk on your lunch break. Whatever you choose for your exercise pattern, make it fit into your daily schedule so you can sustain it over the long term.

People vary in how they like to exercise. Some like to work out alone. I read the newspaper while riding on the exercise bike so I can kill two birds with one stone. Others choose exercise classes or prefer to walk with friends. There is no reason why you cannot integrate a social aspect into your exercise, especially if it helps you maintain your exercise regimen. Finally, if you do not think you are getting all the benefits you should with your exercise routine, ask a professional for help. Meet with a personal trainer, explain your goals, and develop a program that will work for you. Whatever you do, develop an exercise program.

4

CALORIES IN, CALORIES OUT

WE HAVE NOW REVIEWED the role of exercise and genetics in the obesity problem. There is one more fundamental concept that people need to understand before we review many of the popular diets. I refer to this concept as "calories in, calories out."

Your body is basically a reservoir. Every day you take in a number of calories and you expend a certain number of calories. If you take in more calories than you expend, the surplus calories are usually stored as body fat. If you expend more calories than you take in, you make up the extra calories needed, usually by depleting your body fat. People can take in more calories by eating more food, especially if they eat energy-rich foods high in sugar and fat. You can expend more calories through exercise. This concept is illustrated in Table 3.

Your body is a reservoir that reflects your net calorie intake and output over the years. It is no different from a reservoir of water that has streams flowing into it and streams flowing out of it. The water level will rise and fall based on inflow and outflow. If you bought this book with the goal of long-term weight loss, you need to stand in front of the mirror and recognize that your current body weight is the result of your present diet and exercise pattern. To achieve long-term sustained weight loss, you will need to change your diet

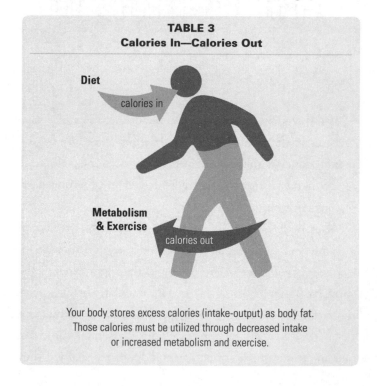

TABLE 3
Calories In—Calories Out

Diet

calories in

Metabolism
& Exercise

calories out

Your body stores excess calories (intake-output) as body fat.
Those calories must be utilized through decreased intake
or increased metabolism and exercise.

or change your exercise pattern to adjust your body fat. As we noted in the last chapter, weight loss can be achieved by modulating either diet or exercise. The greatest benefit, however, occurs if you change *both* diet and exercise. This is no different from the reservoir analogy. The greatest change in the water level in the reservoir will occur if we decrease inflow and increase outflow.

It is unfortunate that many people hope that some simple miracle pill will cure their weight problem. It is even more disturbing to see frequent advertisements on TV or in the newspaper advocating some herbal or vitamin-based "cure" that will melt your fat away while you sleep. People can use medications such as amphetamines, or hormones such as thyroxine, for the purpose of weight loss. These drugs increase your metabolic rate, but with the risk of short- and long-term medical problems. No natural agent available in the marketplace will turn your body into a thermonuclear reactor at night and melt away your body fat. As long as we are debunking myths, I will also tell you that there is no tooth fairy and that Santa Claus did not leave your presents under the Christmas tree.

The long-term key to a successful weight-control effort is through a combination of diet and exercise. The extra calories stored in your body are the result of relative overeating and must be burned off through calorie expenditure. Your body has been designed by nature to give up those calories only if it needs to. You cannot fight thousands of years of evolution. Once you accept that concept, it is much easier to move on.

5

THE DIET SPECTRUM

THE AMERICAN PUBLIC may have an obesity problem, but it is not for lack of popular diets. A wide spectrum of diets are available, and each is considerably different. Which one is best is certainly becoming a topic of national prominence in part due to the obesity epidemic. I would like to put the different types of diets into perspective for you.

Most diets are referred to by name or a number ratio. Table 4 (see page 24) illustrates a spectrum of diets representative of those that are available to the American public. Any diet can be classified by its macronutrient components. Macronutrients are carbohydrate, protein, and fat. If you name the diet, I will tell you where it fits in the table. Some

TABLE 4
Comparing Low-Carbohydrate Diets
with Recommended Diets

	Low-Carbohydrate Diets		
	Atkins	**Protein Power**	**Sugar Busters**
Total daily calories (kcal)	1,600	1,600	1,600
Carbohydrates (g)	22 (5%)***	33 (8%)	162 (40%)
Protein (g)	146 (35%)	149 (35%)	113 (28%)
Fat (g)	104 (59%)	97 (53%)	55 (32%)
Saturated fat (g)	47 (26%)	33 (19%)	17 (9%)
Cholesterol (mg)	924	657	280
Dietary fiber (g)	4	11	24

*ADA, American Diabetes Association
**AHA, American Heart Association

diets, such as the South Beach diet or the Atkins diet, even vary where they fit based on what phase of the diet you are in.

When a diet is referred to by its individual components, it will have three percentages, such as 40-30-30. The first number is the percentage of total calories that come from carbohydrate. The second percentage is that of total calories from protein. The third number is the percentage of total calories from fat. For example, in the American Heart Association diet, more than 55 percent of the total calories come from carbohydrate, less than 30 percent from protein, and 15 percent from fat. The Zone diet, in contrast, has 40 percent of its total calories from carbohydrate, roughly 30 percent from protein, and 30 percent from fat.

	Recommended Diets	
Zone	ADA* Exchange	AHA**
1,600	1,600	1,600
170 (40%)	240 (60%)	220 (>55%)
120 (28%)	82 (20%)	28–72 (12–18%)
49 (32%)	35 (20%)	53 (>30%)
12 (7%)	11 (6%)	18 (<10%)
264	112	<300
18	22	>25

***Percentage of total daily calorie intake
Source: *Cleveland Clinic Journal of Medicine,* Vol. 68, p. 765, Sept. 2001.

An important point to understand is the difference in energy levels from the different food groups. Fat has the highest energy content at 9 calories per gram, carbohydrate at 5 calories per gram, and protein at 4 calories per gram. Thus, even though the amount of fat and protein calories may be the same in a diet based on total caloric percentages, you would take in twice as much protein on a weight basis due to its lower energy content.

As you look at the various diets, there are some interesting comparisons. The first is that the amount of protein and fat as a percentage of total calories tends to be equal. The diets vary by their carbohydrate percentages. You might ask, "What is a low-carbohydrate diet?" In the press and medical literature, "low-carbohydrate" is defined as anything less than the carbohydrate content of the American Heart Association diet. I believe that this is problematic because the Zone diet, which is 40-30-30, has roughly 65 percent of the carbohydrate content of the American Heart Association diet but 400 percent of the carbohydrate content of the Atkins diet. A number of diets use the 40-30-30 ratio. The Zone diet may be the most well known, but other diets such as Sugar Busters, Prism, and Weight Watchers have somewhat similar calorie percentages. So what is low-carbohydrate?

Dieticians have a more appropriate way of classifying the various diets. Dieticians would consider a diet with less than 10 percent of calories from carbohydrate as "low carbohydrate." That would include the early phases of the South Beach diet, or the Atkins diet. Diets such as the Zone diet, with 40 percent carbohydrate, would be considered "moderate" carbohydrate. The American Heart Association diet would be termed "high" carbohydrate. I believe the American public has been confused by referring to all diets with less carbohydrate than the American Heart Association as "low carbohydrate."

My initial experiences in learning about these diets preceded my desire to counsel patients. I was interested at that time in losing weight myself. I initially started the process several years ago when I followed the American Heart Association diet and gained weight. I also gave up red meat and gained weight. What ultimately worked for me was moving from the percentages recommended by the American Heart

Association diet to the 40-30-30 area. I have subsequently maintained that nutritional balance and have not had any problems maintaining my weight over time.

The diet that is not addressed in Table 4 is a vegetarian diet, which actually has the highest percentage of carbohydrate at 80 percent of total calories. That is in part because it is hard to find protein sources, without eating meat or fish, that do not have high amounts of carbohydrate in them. Interestingly, I had noted for years that my patients who became vegetarians tended to gain weight. Initially, I found that perplexing, but now I understand the mechanism. Vegetarians have to consume a lot of carbohydrate to get adequate protein intake.

The observations I am going to make about the various diets are personal observations. I have not subjected these observations to randomized trials to prove them. I have, however, watched my patients for years and I can tell you what has worked for them and what has worked for me as well. I will also note that I do not think there is an ideal diet for everyone. Each individual is unique. They all have their own likes and dislikes as far as food groups are concerned, and they all have different exercise levels and genetic backgrounds. That said, I do believe that every diet has some good features as well as some problems.

The Atkins diet certainly is one of the most well known. Since Dr. Atkins published his first book in 1972,[8] there has been a tremendous controversy as to the role of dietary fat and carbohydrate. Dr. Atkins has often been dismissed as a renegade by the medical community. The success of the Atkins diet is in large part due to its markedly restricted carbohydrate intake. Many people have been able to lose weight with the Atkins diet; I believe that if you can lose weight with this diet and have not had a significant rise in your serum cholesterol, it certainly is a reasonable program for you to follow.

However, several problems are associated with the Atkins diet. The first problem to consider is using the Atkins diet in conjunction with athletic activities. The Atkins diet, by its nature, causes the body to reduce its stored sugar levels. These stored sugars, in the form of glycogen, are often utilized while the body is exercising. Patients of mine who have used the Atkins diet tended to have a significant drop in their energy level associated with exercise. It is, however, a reasonable diet for people who lead a sedentary lifestyle or have sedentary job activity.

The other major concern I have always had with the Atkins diet is what exactly happens to a patient's cholesterol level. Some people who follow this diet, because of their heavy consumption of fat, can have a rise in cholesterol levels. This is an adverse effect for my cardiac patients, and the diet is not acceptable in that regard. Finally, although some people can lose a considerable amount of weight on the Atkins diet in spite of eating a high proportion of dietary fat, the basic concept of calories in, calories out still applies. People taking in calories in the form of fat are taking in 9 calories per gram. If the same people who lose weight consuming one-half pound of bacon per day changed their dietary intake to one-quarter pound of turkey, they would get nearly the same amount of protein but dramatically less fat. That would promote faster weight loss and also a reduction in blood fat levels.

The South Beach diet by Dr. Arthur Agatston has many similarities to the Atkins diet. Both start with at least several weeks of severe carbohydrate restriction. Ultimately the South Beach diet and the Atkins diet want you to increase your carbohydrate intake over time to a point that allows you to maintain long-term weight control. For most people, this involves moving into some type of eating program that would be more typically found in the moderate carbohydrate levels of 30 to 40 percent of total calories. The South Beach diet does, however, offer some significant improvements to the previous Atkins concepts.

The South Beach diet tends to be far less restrictive in salads and vegetables than the Atkins diet. The South Beach diet also promotes favoring fat sources that are high in omega-3 fatty acids, such as fish. It also suggests getting fat from plant sources, such as peanuts and almonds. By using those sources of fat, you are less likely to have a rise in your cholesterol and might actually have a significant improvement in your HDL, or "good" cholesterol. Finally, the South Beach diet appears to have a more concrete transition into long-term weight control. Some people who try to follow the Atkins program fail to make the transition into a long-term successful eating program. I believe that several factors are probably involved in that failure, but the South Beach diet appears to have more concrete advice and practical suggestions in how to make that transition. I believe that because of the changes in fat and protein sources, as well as the improvement in the transition steps, the South Beach diet represents a significant improvement over the Atkins diet.

The Zone diet is promoted by Dr. Barry Sears, and I believe that it is the most nutritionally balanced for the majority of my patients and probably for the majority of Americans. The Zone diet promotes a calorie intake of 40-30-30. I propose that the majority of Americans would be able to achieve weight control following the recommended Zone ratios shown in Table 4. Just like many other genetic attributes, I believe our ability to consume carbohydrate is probably a bell-shaped curve. I suspect the peak of the bell curve is between 40 and 50 percent carbohydrate intake, with the smaller aspects of the bell stretching out to 70 to 80 percent carbohydrate on the right and possibly down to 20 percent carbohydrate on the left. That is, some people can consume 70 to 80 percent carbohydrate without gaining any weight; others, even if they consume only 30 percent carbohydrate, will gain weight. Where you are on the bell-shaped curve is determined in part by your genetics and further manipulated by your exercise pattern.

I strongly recommend a Zone-style diet, or a 40-30-30, for people who are interested in athletic performance. I routinely recommend it to my friends who compete in athletics, whether golf or triathlons. I previously recommended the diet to my patients and still do on occasion. The major downfall of the Zone diet for many of my patients is the necessity to measure food, weigh food, and use a calculator. Although some people ultimately need to resort to those techniques because of difficulty in achieving weight loss, I believe that most people who try an exercise and diet program are able to lose weight without having to do more than read labels on the food they eat. Ultimately, I derived the three principles covered in the next chapter because of my patients' frustrations in applying the principles of the Zone diet.

Weight Watchers is an excellent program. I have a fondness in my heart for Weight Watchers because my mother was always able to achieve success through it. Anything that made Mom happy made the Gavin boys happy. My brothers and I actually grew up in part eating Weight Watchers–approved menus. Weight Watchers is an excellent program for people who need a group support mechanism. It does, however, involve meetings and fees and uses a calorie-counting mechanism called points. Many of my patients were not interested in following that kind of structured program. I should note that the majority of my patients are male, and Weight Watchers tends to be a female-dominated organization. If Weight Watchers works for you, it is a great program.

The American Heart Association diet is relatively high in carbohydrates and low in fat. This diet was designed to promote low cholesterol levels, not weight loss. Even though it is low in fat, it can be high in energy, and those calories are very easily converted to fat within the body. The American Heart Association diet and the USDA Food Guide Pyramid shown in Table 5 (see page 32) both obtain a relatively high percentage of their calories through carbohydrate. Some of my patients can tolerate a diet like that; however, in my opin-

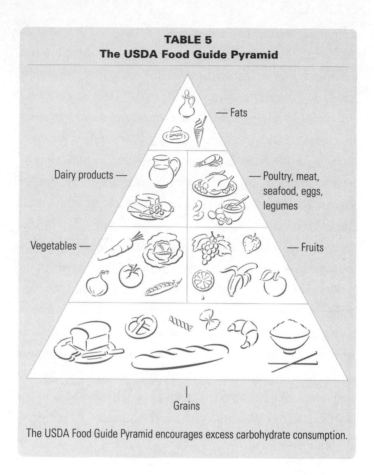

TABLE 5
The USDA Food Guide Pyramid

— Fats

Dairy products —

— Poultry, meat, seafood, eggs, legumes

Vegetables —

— Fruits

Grains

The USDA Food Guide Pyramid encourages excess carbohydrate consumption.

ion the majority seem to gain weight. A very simple question to ask yourself is, "Have I been following the American Heart Association diet and gaining weight?" If you have been gaining weight, then this is probably not the right diet for you.

I have also seen a very unfortunate diet approach that you should be aware of. Some people, frustrated with their inability to lose weight on the standard American Diabetes Association diet or the American Heart Association diet, jump all the way to the Atkins diet and are often able to lose significant amounts of weight. Unfortunately, they then return to their former eating habits and regain the weight they lost. This cycle of weight gain and weight loss becomes relentless and demoralizing. These people should move themselves long-term into a 40-30-30 program and stay there.

As I noted earlier, there is no perfect diet. Each diet seems to have its strong points and also its weak points. I do think it is helpful to try to consider what type of diet you are eating now and what the relative proportions of the various food groups are. As you try to deal with weight loss, it seems to be helpful to lower carbohydrate intake and especially starch intake. Move to the diets more to the left in Table 4 of where you are now. Increasing your exercise level will also help you lose weight. If you are gaining weight and eating in a given range of carbohydrate percentage and are already doing a reasonable exercise program, then I believe it is even more important to cut down the carbohydrate intake in your diet.

6

THE THREE-RULE DIET

SINCE MY PATIENTS BECAME frustrated by trying to follow the somewhat complicated diets out there, I decided to try to simplify these programs into something easier to follow. My patients wanted a plan that didn't require a calculator, a food scale, or numerous trips to specialty or health food stores. They wanted something easy to follow, with rules they could remember and still live a normal life.

So here is the Three-Rule Diet. You won't have to weigh or measure food on a regular basis with this diet, but you will need to be aware of what you are eating.

Rule #1: Eat Three Meals a Day

I know that seems very simple, but many of my patients skip breakfast or lunch, and some patients in my practice formerly ate only one meal per day—dinner. The effect of eating a large number of calories at the end of your day has been studied in animals but not in humans. Rats that are fed three equal-calorie meals throughout the day tend to have a normal body weight. Rats that are fed the same total calories as one large meal at the end of the day are fat.

The important point is that eating the majority of your calorie intake late in the day is associated with obesity. That occurs even if you are eating an appropriate amount of calories per day. A recent survey showed that skipping breakfast is a marker for obesity and diabetes. If you want to skip a meal, skip dinner. The simplest diet I know is not to eat after 4:00 in the afternoon. I have known people to adopt this principle and have successful weight loss over the long term, but it is a very difficult style of eating to follow for various social and physical reasons.

I stress the importance of breakfast and lunch, because people who skip breakfast or lunch tend to overeat at night. These people starve themselves throughout the day, and then when they get home begin consuming large amounts of food. I have one patient who ate only one meal a day—dinner—and now eats two meals a day. She eats breakfast and lunch, and is no longer hungry enough to eat dinner. She has lost considerable weight. If you have a difficult time eating breakfast, either because of habit or time constraints, I recommend that you try eating peanut butter on a piece of toast. Peanut butter on toast is an excellent breakfast option. The combination of peanut butter and toast gives a relatively good balance between carbohydrate, protein, and fat. It is also quick and easy to make. By eating breakfast you fire up your metabolic engine and make it easier for your body to burn excess fat.

Rule #2:
Eat Some Lean Protein with Every Meal

This is often one of the more difficult rules to adopt. The challenge is to define what type of lean protein you like. The protein source can be meat, fish, fowl, or even peanut butter. If it is a vegetable source such as peanut butter or soynut butter, you need to ensure that it has at least 7 to 8 grams of protein per serving. Many types of lean protein sources are available, but what is very important is that it has to be a protein source that you like. Examples of lean protein include egg whites, peanut butter, smoked fish, Canadian bacon, lean lunchmeat, nonfat yogurt, low-fat cottage cheese, and mozzarella cheese, not to mention multiple types of meat, fish, and fowl.

I stress to my patients the need to eat lean protein because it will keep you from getting hungry between meals. Of the various food groups, protein is the most effective in curbing your hunger. Fat intake can slow your digestion and provide some benefit in controlling hunger. Carbohydrate is proba-

Lean (Low-Fat) Protein Options
egg whites, 2–3
smoked fish, lox
natural peanut butter, 2 Tbsp*
Canadian bacon, 2 slices
turkey bacon, 2 slices
low-fat or nonfat cottage cheese
string cheese, 1–2 sticks
nonfat yogurt, flavored
deli meats, turkey, ham, or roast beef
tuna, 6 oz
beef, favor top round, sirloin, filet, tri-tip, and London broil
chicken, remove skin after cooking
turkey, remove skin after cooking
fish, any kind
pork, favor tenderloin, or pork chops without the bone and fat trimmed
wild game, elk, venison

*Peanut butter is acceptable as the fats are unsaturated and may improve your HDL (good cholesterol).

bly the least effective food for providing satiety. I ask my patients to do a simple experiment. One morning, have two pieces of toast or a bagel for breakfast. You can put on them all the jam or marmalade you want. Write down on a piece of paper how many hours after breakfast you get hungry. The next morning, have one piece of toast or half a bagel for breakfast, but put peanut butter on it. You will find that you will not get hungry for an additional two hours. I have experienced this effect personally.

When I was heavy, I used to eat a bagel for breakfast at roughly 6:00 in the morning. I would get to the hospital and start work by 7:00, and often by 8:30 or 9:00 I would be hungry. As I was walking through the doctors' lounge at 8:30 or 9:00, I would pass a plate of doughnuts and pastries and pick one up. I was, after all, hungry. Now that I eat lean protein with my breakfast every morning, I walk by the same plate of doughnuts but I have no interest in them. If you eat lean protein with your meal, you will not be hungry for an additional two to three hours. I have found that it is very easy not to eat if you are not hungry. The converse is also true: It is very difficult to continue to avoid food when you are hungry, and the food choices people make for snacking are often poor. I believe that a major problem of high-carbohydrate, low-protein diets is that they make people excessively hungry between meals.

Rule #3: No White at Night

Patients often look at me a little confused after I tell them this rule. I want you to think about what is white. *No White at Night* means no rice, bread, potatoes, or pasta. It also applies to all the colored variants of those foods. Also banned at your evening meal would be red potatoes, brown rice, whole-wheat bread, and starchy vegetables such as corn, which I might note comes in a white variety! Dinner should become lean meat, fish, or fowl and all the salad and vegetables you want. I would also suggest that you not use table sugar and avoid milk at dinner as well.

You might be thinking, "Why do we need to limit starch intake?" Starch is, after all, a low-fat food group. When we send cattle to Nebraska to fatten them up, what do we feed them? The stockyards feed those animals low-fat grain. Those cattle are mammals just like us. The cattle producers do not feed the animals lard, nor do they feed them vegetable oil. Yet those same animals dramatically increase their fat content. In Lewis County, south of my hometown, the local hog producers feed their hogs old bread purchased from the Safeway stores. There is *NO* fat in a loaf of bread. The hogs, also mammals, add to their body fat by eating the bread.

The explanation for the conversion process of sugar to fat is efficiency. Our bodies do not store significant amounts of energy in sugar. The body does have some sugar stores, called glycogen, which are located in the liver to supply the brain with sugar in emergencies, and also in the muscles to be burned if the fight-or-flight system is activated. The majority of our energy stores are in body fat.

A kilogram (2.2 pounds) of glycogen has 5,000 calories. A kilogram of body fat has 9,000 calories. In the same weight, the body is able to carry nearly twice the stored energy in fat than it can in sugar. A significant reason for this is that fat is relatively dehydrated. The stored glycogen has water with it so that it can be burned immediately in times of emergency.

For example, if I were to give you a thousand pennies, how would you carry those pennies around? I would suspect that by the end of the day, those pennies would be converted into ten paper bills. That would be a much more efficient way for you to carry that money. Your body is basically doing the same thing. Your body converts any excess sugar calories to fat within twenty-four hours.

A concept that should not be forgotten here is that you can get fat eating nonfat foods. Just like hogs and cattle, humans can gain weight and store body fat on a diet that is high in carbohydrate. As you walk through a supermarket, you will be inundated with bright, colorful labels touting low-fat or reduced-fat foods. Nonfat foods can still be loaded with energy in the form of carbohydrate. Although that food source may go through your mouth as no fat, your body will not store it that way.

All food sources are broken down into a universal energy source and then ideally stored as body fat if the body has excess calories. It is relatively straightforward and easy for the body to store the energy of carbohydrate or fat that is taken orally. It is more difficult for the body to store protein calories as body fat. The process of breaking down protein to a simple energy source has a significant energy consumption, and the net return in storing protein calories as fat is not very efficient for the body. Do not, however, assume that eating protein will build your muscles. Eating protein allows you to have additional calories that you can burn for energy. To build your muscles you must exercise and consume protein at the same time.

Another important point is the need to drink large amounts of water. The human body needs at least 1 liter of water per day. Most nutritional programs recommend that you drink eight large glasses of water per day. This is certainly reasonable. Remember, your body is predominantly water. If you are trying to burn body fat, you need to drink even more water.

As noted earlier, a kilogram of body fat contains 9,000 calories. If you were in a starvation mode, you could live for nine days on that amount of calories. To adequately burn that fat requires adding at least a liter of water per day. Thus, to burn 2.2 pounds of fat, you need to consume nearly 20 pounds of water. Stored body fat is an extremely efficient, light source of energy that can be unlocked with adequate amounts of water.

A good rule is to try to balance the calories between your three meals throughout the day. If your diet is going to consist of 1,800 calories, have roughly 400 to 500 calories at every meal. Depending on what time you eat dinner, you may note that you begin to get hungry at 4:00 or 5:00. If you know that your dinner is going to be late, try to have some type of snack that has a significant protein content between 4:00 and 5:00 in the afternoon. In Chapter Nine, we will give you some very practical examples of what sorts of food you can eat at various meals. If you want to slant your calorie intake toward one part of the day or another, slant your largest meal to be breakfast and your smallest meal to be dinner.

There is an old saying among people who counsel dieters: "Eat breakfast like a king, lunch like a storekeeper, and dinner like a pauper." By consuming the majority of your calories early in the day, you have the greatest opportunity to burn them off. By delaying your calorie intake to the latter part of the day, you give your body the greatest opportunity to store the extra calories. If you make the evening meal high in starches such as rice, bread, and pasta, you further drive the hormonal mechanisms of the body to store those calories as fat. Those hormonal mechanisms are mediated by insulin, and the foods that you are being asked to restrict have a very high glycemic index.

By reducing the starch in your diet you will change the glycemic index of the foods you are eating. The glycemic index of food groups is probably important to all people trying to lose weight, and especially to diabetics. The glycemic index of a given food group is a measurement of how fast your blood sugar rises after you eat that food group. The faster your blood sugar rises, the higher the glycemic index of that particular food.[9] The food with the highest glycemic index would be sugar in water. Potatoes, white bread, and rice have a very high glycemic index. Foods with a high glycemic index produce a very high insulin response within your body. That insulin rise ultimately leads to hypoglycemia and hunger. In addition, insulin is the primary hormone in driving production of body fat from excess calories. Changing the carbohydrate in your diet at night from starch such as rice, bread, and potatoes to vegetables or salad reduces your insulin level and may help promote weight loss.

Another important concept to understand in conjunction with the glycemic index is glycemic load. Glycemic load is the measurement of the total carbohydrate or sugar in a given food group. Food groups may have a high glycemic index but a low amount of total carbohydrate or glycemic load. For example, potatoes have a high glycemic index and also a high glycemic load. Thus, the rise in your blood sugar after eating a meal with potatoes will be relatively high and sustained.

Carrots have a high glycemic index, nearly as high as that of potatoes. Carrots, however, have a low glycemic load. The potential spike that can be produced in your blood sugar from eating a certain amount of carrots may be sharp, but it will not be particularly prolonged. That is why some people consider carrots *bad* in your diet when trying to lose weight. In reality, the glycemic load of carrots is so low that they are not a particular problem. You will not get fat by eating carrots.

In the public press you will often see the glycemic index of various food groups. Unfortunately, you will not often see the glycemic load of those same food groups, which is really the most important piece of information. I do believe that eating a low-glycemic-index diet will help you lose weight. Eating low-glycemic-index foods will decrease your insulin levels, and that should make it easier for you to lose weight. Many books have been written about the concept of glycemic index and how it can affect weight loss. A good reference is *The New Glucose Revolution* by Jennie Brand-Miller.[10]

Table 6 (see page 46) shows the glycemic index and glycemic load of some common foods. It is important to note that the more processed the food becomes, the higher its glycemic index tends to be. For example, orange juice has a higher glycemic index than plain oranges because the fiber has been broken down. It is also important to note that some foods such as brown rice and white rice have varying glycemic indices but significant glycemic loads. Finally, I would again like to draw your attention to carrots. Carrots have a relatively high glycemic index, but you will note that their glycemic load is low. You would need to eat a pound and a half of raw carrots to get the same glycemic load as an English muffin.

A good research tool for learning more about the glycemic index and glycemic load of various food groups is the Internet. If you search the Internet for "glycemic index" you will find several sites that list hundreds of food groups. A particularly good Web site is www.glycemicindex.com, which is maintained by the University of Sydney in Australia. It offers excellent information and listings of food. I would especially urge you, if you are diabetic, to learn more about low-glycemic-index foods and favor them in your diet.

In my own diet, I have definitely moved to lower-glycemic-index foods. I eat less starch such as bagels or pastries in the morning. I also rarely eat rice, bread, or potatoes anymore at night. Instead of eating starch at night I eat carbohydrate in the form of vegetables, either cooked or in a salad. I have reduced not only my glycemic index but also my glycemic load. Although I cannot *prove* that this has made a difference in my weight, I will note that my body fat is the lowest it has been in twenty years, and I believe it has made a significant difference in my ability not only to lose weight but also to maintain my present weight. Ironically, I used to believe that the problem with the baked potato was the extras like butter or sour cream that you put on it. Now I believe the potato is just as big a problem as the extras.

Patients also ask me how much lean protein is enough. I ask patients to eat *reasonable* quantities of lean protein. A rule of thumb might be to eat a number of grams of protein as high as 50 percent of your weight in pounds. So, if you weigh

	TABLE 6		
	Glycemic Index and Glycemic Load of Common Foods		
Food	**Glycemic Index* (glucose = 100)**	**Glycemic Load****	**Serving Size**
Orange juice	57	15	250 cc
Oranges	31	12	250 cc
Apple juice	40	12	250 cc
Apples	40	6	120 cc
Grapefruit	25	3	120 g
Peaches	28	4	120 g
Pears	28	4	120 g
Grapes	43	7	120 g
Raisins	64	28	60 g
Watermelon	72	4	120 g
Bananas	51	13	120 g
Mango	41	8	120 g
Pineapple	51	8	120 g
Plums	24	3	120 g
Strawberries	40	1	120 g
Brown rice	50	16	150 g
White rice	56	24	150 g
White potato—baked	85	26	150 g
White potato—boiled	58	16	150 g
White potato—mashed	91	18	150 g
Whole-grain pasta	32	14	180 g
Sweet corn	60	20	150 g

Food	Glycemic Index* (glucose = 100)	Glycemic Load**	Serving Size
Carrots	47	3	80 g
Couscous	65	23	150 g
Fettucine	35	15	180 g
Macaroni	45	22	180 g
White bread	70	10	30 g
Rye bread	41	5	30 g
Bagel	72	25	70 g
Whole-wheat bread	52	10	30 g
Buckwheat bread	47	10	30 g
French baguette	95	15	30 g
Kaiser roll	73	12	30 g

*Glycemic index: less than 55 is low.
**Glycemic load: less than 10 is low.

160 pounds, you can eat up to 80 grams of protein per day. If you are very athletic, you may need to increase your protein intake to 1 gram of protein per pound. You certainly do not need to consume more protein than that. Most obese patients I see are not consuming adequate protein. By eating lean protein at every meal, including breakfast, my average patient probably increases his or her overall protein intake. At your evening meal, a chicken breast or 4 to 6 ounces of fish or meat is more than adequate. I now find it ironic that when I go out to a restaurant that specializes in steak, I usually order the "petite filet," which is often 8 ounces and the

smallest steak on the menu. An excellent visual cue is to choose a lean protein portion that is the size of the palm of your hand. That amount of protein should be more than adequate for most adults. If you are a young adult and engage in strenuous exercise, you could probably increase that.

Fruits are high in fiber and vitamins and are a good supplement to any diet. However, you should restrict your intake of fruit juices. Avoid orange juice, because it is high in sugar, and also fruits that are high in sugar and release their sugar very fast into the bloodstream. These fruits have a high glycemic index or load. They include grapes, raisins, oranges, peaches, nectarines, and tangerines. Pears and apples should be favored, as they have a lower glycemic index or load, and the sugar will be released more slowly into the bloodstream due to the fiber content. Whenever possible, always eat the whole fruit and avoid fruit juices, even from fruit such as apples. By eating the whole fruit, you get more vitamins and fiber; the whole fruit will definitely have a lower glycemic index or load.

I encourage patients to restrict their starch intake to the equivalent of one slice of bread at breakfast and lunch. That starch can be in any number of forms, such as an English muffin, half a bagel, or a bowl of oatmeal. Choose breads or cereals that are not refined, whole-grain products, stone-ground products, and oatmeal, and avoid products based on white flour. By doing this you will increase the fiber content in your diet and reduce the initial sugar load that your body experiences after a meal. When they change their diet in this way, many people, myself included, find that they no longer become sleepy after a meal. My energy level is relatively constant for 4 to 5 hours, and I no longer get hungry 2 to 3 hours after eating.

How do I know I did something wrong at a meal?

- IF YOU'RE HUNGRY within 2 hours after eating, you didn't have enough protein.
- IF YOU'RE SLEEPY after a meal, you had too many starchy carbs.

A simple guideline to follow with your meals is the following. If you are hungry two hours after eating, your meal had an inadequate amount of protein. If you are sleepy an hour or two after eating your meal, then you consumed too much carbohydrate at that meal. Note the effects of the foods you eat have on you after you have eaten, and make appropriate changes based on how you feel. A well-balanced meal should allow you to be alert and hunger-free for at least 3 or 4 hours.

I have asked you with these three rules to limit the amount of starch in your diet. I have also limited the amount of fat in your diet by asking you to eat lean protein sources (see the list on page 38). I will not restrict the amount of vegetables or salad in your diet. You can eat unlimited amounts of nonstarchy vegetables and unlimited amounts of salad with this diet. There is carbohydrate or sugar in vegetables, but it is so interwoven with fiber that it is released relatively slowly and the amount of sugar is not that great. Granted, there is more sugar in carrots than celery, but I have never known anyone who has gotten fat eating carrots. So, regardless of the meal, you can eat as much salad or vegetables as you choose.

Patients often ask about the use of salad dressing. This clearly is a source of dietary fat intake. Find a low-fat or even nonfat salad dressing that you like. Try to use salad dressings that have a significant amount of vinegar content. Favor salad dressings that use olive oil. If your major fat intake at night is in the form of salad dressing, you will have markedly restricted your fat intake by making these adjustments.

The same hormone system involved in breaking down your body's fat, which is mediated by a hormone called glucagon, is also responsible for breaking down the dietary fat that you are eating at night. There is significant controversy in the medical literature about what is the right amount of fat for people to consume. It may be that consuming a small but reasonable amount of fat is helpful in keeping your fat-burning system activated and primed.

Patients often ask me if it is allowable to drink alcoholic beverages such as wine or hard liquor on this diet. It is important to note that alcoholic beverages have a significant carbohydrate load. All the calories in alcoholic beverages are in the form of carbohydrate. Table 7, showing some alcoholic beverages and their caloric content, appears on page 51. Two glasses of wine is fundamentally equal to a large baked potato. For the purpose of weight loss, complete abstinence from alcohol is probably ideal. If you do choose to drink a

TABLE 7 Common Alcoholic Beverages				
	Amount	**Calories**	**Protein**	**Carbs**
Beer	12 oz	146	1	13
Light Beer	12 oz	99	1	5
Ultra Light	12 oz	95	.6	2.6
O'Doul's	12 oz	70	1.2	13.3
Wine, Red	4 oz	92	0	2
White	4 oz	82	0	2
Whiskey	1 oz	64	0	0
Vodka	1 oz	64	0	0
Gin	1 oz	64	0	0
Tequila	1 oz	65	0	0
Margarita	7 oz	160	0	24
Daiquiri	7 oz	210	0	35
Bloody Mary	7 oz	104	1	4
Pina Colada	7 oz	260	1	37
Tonic	6 oz	64	0	16
Diet Tonic	6 oz	2	0	1

It is important to note that most alcoholic beverages have significant calories but do not raise blood sugar like fruit juices. The higher caloric options in this table do have significant carbohydrate content in addition to alcohol.

limited amount of alcohol while actively dieting, then you will need to either increase your exercise or acknowledge that your weight loss may be slower over time.

I actually encourage many of my patients with cardiovascular disease to drink half a glass of red wine in the evening. When I was actively trying to lose weight, that was the amount of wine that I would consume. Once you have achieved your weight-loss target, you can then consider increasing your starch intake or your alcohol intake. A very reasonable approach is to consume your carbohydrate as an alcoholic beverage at dinnertime. That may be 1 to 2 mixed drinks or 1 to 2 glasses of wine. In the past, a relatively popular diet referred to as "the drinking man's diet" promoted restricting starches other than alcohol in the evening.

Patients also ask me if they need to take a multivitamin. Most people following the Three-Rule Diet will actually increase their vegetable intake. It certainly is reasonable to consider consuming a one-a-day adult multivitamin. Also consider reviewing your common foodstuffs during the day. If you eat a diet that is relatively low in milk or other dairy products, you may also want to consider using a calcium supplement. Other than an adult multivitamin and calcium supplementation, it is unlikely that most people will need additional vitamins. If you believe in using additional vitamin supplements, that is acceptable. The added vitamins will probably not harm you, and you can decide the benefit versus the cost.

More important than vitamins is how dieting may affect your medications. The foods favored by the diet should not affect your medications, but your weight loss will. Your need for medications for high blood pressure, diabetes, and high cholesterol may decrease dramatically with weight loss. As your weight drops, check your blood pressure more frequently, and check with your doctor about decreasing your medications. If you have diabetes, be sure to read Chapter Eight. Dealing with the need to decrease your medications is a good problem to have.

A common problem for some of my patients is trying to figure out how their daily work schedule meshes with these dietary principles. If you have irregular sleep hours or work a graveyard shift, I propose the following. After awakening from what is your normal sleep time, consider your first meal to be your breakfast meal. It is quite appropriate to consume some starch with that meal. You still need to follow the other principles and also consume some lean protein at that meal. At the last meal of your "day," before you sleep, consume no starch. Consider that meal to be your supper meal. That meal should consist of some lean protein and, again, all the salad or vegetables you want.

It is important to recognize how much protein or carbohydrate you might be eating in a given meal, but the good news is that you simply need to read. Because of government regulations, most of the foods you eat, with the exception of vegetables and fruits, come labeled with the number of calories in a given serving, further categorized by the number of calories from carbohydrate, fat, and protein. By simply looking at the box of cereal or the container of yogurt, you quickly will find out the calories and the breakdown of the foods you are eating.

In summary, then, I recommend that you follow three

simple principles in your eating: Eat three meals per day, consume a reasonable portion of lean protein with every meal, and, finally, eat no white (starch) at night. Try to consume no more than the equivalent of one slice of bread at breakfast and lunch. Eat all the salad and nonstarchy vegetables that you choose. Finally, increase your consumption of water and fruits and try to limit juices. If you apply these principles to foods that you like, you should find the changes in your diet relatively simple. I developed these rules to help people achieve weight loss in a simple way, and I am happy to say that when patients return and have lost weight, they commonly tell me, "It's not that hard." I believe you can do it, too.

When a patient comes to my office I give them my instructions for exercise and the three rules of the diet written on a prescription blank. I do that to emphasize my belief that their diet and exercise pattern is as important as any medication I may prescribe. I ask them to put the prescription on their refrigerator door. At the back of this book on page 172, you will find *your* prescription. Place it on your refrigerator door, and follow it.

7

LONG-TERM WEIGHT CONTROL

T HE SUCCESS OF ANY DIET or weight-loss program should
not be measured in short-term weight loss, but long-
term weight control. You may be able to reach your target
weight loss over the next three to six months by following
the Three-Rule Diet, but what is most important to me is
that you keep your weight off over time. Many people lose
a considerable amount of weight only to slowly gain it back
over time.

Remember, your current body weight is a reflection of
your long-term calorie intake and calorie expenditure. People achieve significant weight loss by increasing their calorie
expenditure over a long period of time and bringing down

their own body fat stores. What is important in the weight-loss process is recognizing what has been the key to your success. People who achieve weight loss by markedly restricting their calorie intake and using a calorie source such as a liquid diet supplement, which deviates from their normal eating and social pattern, are very likely to regain their weight when they return to their old patterns. The more your weight-loss program deviates from what you would normally eat, the more likely you are to regain your weight. I do not perceive myself to be on a diet anymore, but I did significantly change the way I ate several years ago.

Fortunately, for most people, the weight-loss process will take a significant amount of time. In my own case, I lost 10 pounds over one year, and then lost roughly 35 pounds over the next fourteen months. The entire process took more than two years. During that time I discovered foods that I enjoyed eating and a way of eating that kept my energy level high, met my caloric needs, and did not involve getting hungry between meals. I hope that the same thing will happen for you.

A realistic expectation is that someone can lose between 30 and 50 pounds over the course of a year. As noted earlier, body fat has a very high energy content. If you expend, either through increased exercise or by calorie restriction, an extra 325 calories per day, you will lose about 25 pounds over the course of a year. You need to lose more than 650 calories per day to lose 50 pounds per year. Weight loss in excess of 50 pounds per year is very difficult to achieve, except for extremely obese people. Those who weigh more than 350 pounds need significant amounts of muscle mass to support their large body structures. When these people lose weight, they lose not only body fat but also muscle mass. Muscle mass, because of its higher water content, gives greater weight loss. I tell patients that if they can achieve a weight loss of 2 to 4 pounds per month, they are doing quite well.

A core principle of the diet during the period of weight loss is *No White at Night*. When you have reached your target weight, you can begin to reintroduce a limited portion of starch into your supper or evening meal. That may be a small portion of potatoes or rice, or it may be an increased amount of alcohol. Choose low-glycemic-index starches whenever possible, such as brown rice instead of white rice or whole-grain pasta instead of white pasta. Remember, two bottles of beer have the same caloric equivalent as a baked potato.

A reasonable protein portion should be the size of the palm of your hand. That same size is also a reasonable starch portion. When a restaurant serves you a very large baked potato, that potato may actually be three or more starch portions. That lack of understanding of portion control in carbohydrate intake is certainly one of the causes of the obesity epidemic. With whatever starch group you choose to add, add only one, and add it in one reasonable portion.

A registry is maintained in Washington, D.C., for people who have been successful with a weight-loss program and choose to enter it. To be eligible you need to lose 30 pounds and you need to maintain your weight loss for more than one year. I would be eligible for this registry. People in the registry display three important characteristics that should be adopted by anyone seeking long-term weight control: They change the way they eat in the long term. They adopt an exercise program and maintain it. Finally, they monitor their weight in the long term and adjust their diet appropriately. If you want to achieve long-term weight control, I encourage you to adopt these principles as well.

As you make changes in your diet, monitor your weight over the next several weeks and months. Try not to make too many changes in too short a period of time. Typically you should wait at least several weeks to a month to note any changes in your weight. If you are consuming the right amount of calories, your weight will level off and you should be back to a steady state. If your weight begins to rise, then you have added too much starch and you will need to move your eating habits back to those more closely aligned with what you were following when you were losing weight.

The good news is that during your period of weight loss, you will probably discover some foods you like and find that you do not miss those high-energy starches as you thought you would. In my case, I discovered that adding protein to my breakfast kept me from getting hungry until noon. I also learned about yogurt and string cheese from a friend; it is now my standard lunch. By the time you need to deal with weight maintenance versus weight loss, you will be eating in a different way and should have discovered foods that you like and eating patterns that work for you. If you return to your former exercise pattern and also your former eating pattern, you will undoubtedly return to your former weight.

Just as it took several months or even years for you to lose the weight, it will take months and years for you to put the weight back on, but it will return if you return to your prior eating habits. In losing weight you will have discovered what types of foods you can eat and control your weight, but you will not have changed your underlying genetic structure. That will remain with you for life. But you will have the knowledge and power to control your weight if you choose to. In Chapter Nine, I will show you some examples of how I changed my eating at various meals and then how I changed my food intake when I reached my target weight.

8

DIABETES AND WEIGHT LOSS

PEOPLE WITH DIABETES have some unique medical issues involving diet and weight. I have a special empathy for my diabetic patients. My mother is a diabetic. I also have a family history of adult-onset diabetes. Unfortunately, the incidence of diabetes and obesity is going up across the country, and many diabetics seem to have a poor understanding of their illness.

Diabetes is a weight-driven illness. In a recent issue of the *Journal of the American Medical Association*,[11] a survey study showed that the number of obese American adults continues to rise. Not surprisingly, the number of American adults who are diabetic continues to increase in both sexes, all ages, and all races. It is important to understand that diabetes is not a uniform illness. If you have ever known a diabetic child— that is, an individual who had diabetes occur in grade school or high school more than five years ago—I will make a uniform prediction that that individual was thin.

Children with diabetes have a lack of insulin due to some type of autoimmune process in which they destroy their own pancreas. These children cannot make insulin to help control their blood sugar level. Also, they cannot make insulin to help promote storage of body fat. Typically, when these children are diagnosed with new-onset diabetes, they are thin and have just lost a considerable amount of weight. We will call this type of diabetes juvenile-onset, or type 1, diabetes. The diabetes picture in children is getting more complicated, as obese children are now presenting with the type of high insulin levels and diabetes seen in adults and described shortly.

Adults who are diagnosed with diabetes have a much greater diversity in their illness. Most of these adults are overweight. They tend to have normal or even high insulin levels but they have lost sensitivity to the insulin levels in their end-organ tissues, or they simply cannot make enough insulin for the size of their bodies. Adults who develop diabetes in adulthood are commonly referred to as adult-onset diabetics, or type 2 diabetics.

Insulin's role in the body is not only to control blood sugar but also to control body fat. The more body fat one has, the higher the level of insulin required to manage it. The most straightforward way to help a diabetic who is overweight is to help them lose weight. By losing weight, the person can then bring their body size into better balance with the level of insulin that the pancreas can produce.

Patients with diabetes that I meet are often considerably overweight. Commonly they are 20 to 30 percent over their ideal body weight, having at least an extra 40 to 60 pounds of body fat. These individuals are generally referred to me because they have had poor control of their hypertension. Not surprisingly, these patients have all the illnesses attributed to obesity. Besides high blood pressure, they have high cholesterol and possibly underlying cardiovascular disease. When I first talk to these patients I commonly ask them if anyone has ever told them that they should lose weight. The answer is almost always "Yes." I then ask them if anyone has ever told them *how* to lose weight, and the response to that is typically "No." I then ask them two other questions that I think are very important. I ask them if anyone has ever explained to them that if they lose 40 to 60 pounds, their diabetes could go away. The typical response to that question is "No." Finally, I ask them if they were ever on a diabetic diet and gained weight on it. The common response is "Yes."

In Chapter Five, we reviewed the various diets touted to the American public. The diet proposed to most patients by the American Diabetes Association is relatively high in carbohydrate and starch. That diet, in essence, was designed for children who were thin and had relatively insignificant insulin levels. Most adults with adult-onset diabetes are obese, and some of them even have high insulin levels. I believe the majority of Americans would actually gain weight on the

American Diabetes Association diet. I know I would, and I have seen many patients gain weight on this diet.

If you are a diabetic and are following the standard diabetic diet, you are consuming a large amount of your calories as starch and carbohydrate. If you have been gaining weight on this diet, or had difficulty in losing weight on this diet, you need to move your diet toward the left side of Table 4 (see page 24) in the diet spectrum. By reducing your starch and carbohydrate intake, you will probably find it easier to control your blood sugars and you will also find it easier to lose weight. Remember, it is very important to adopt a diet with lower-glycemic-index foods if you are diabetic. That will decrease your need for insulin and help you lose weight.

If you simply have high blood sugar and have been counseled by your doctor to lose weight, you can follow my diet principles, and that should be adequate. If you are diabetic and currently on medication, you will need to work with your doctor toward reducing your medication. If you are diabetic and 40 to 60 pounds overweight and taking only oral medication, you may be able to get rid of your need for medication by losing weight.

What many patients do not understand is that by being on diabetic medication and eating a high-carbohydrate diet, they are actually more inclined to gain weight than to lose weight. Think back to when you initially were diagnosed with diabetes. If you gained weight after your doctor started you on your new medication, then you were eating too much carbohydrate in your diet for your own personal metabolism.

In addition, the medicines can also make people hungry by raising their insulin level. Unfortunately, patients get trapped in a progressive tailspin. They get put on more medication, they get hungrier, they eat more, and they gain more weight. As they gain weight, their blood sugars go up and then they get put on more medication. It is a relentless cycle.

To break the cycle, you need to change your diet. When you reduce your carbohydrate and starch intake, you will first notice that your blood sugars come under better control. If you work with your doctor to reduce your medications, you will find it easier to lose weight. The ultimate goal for any obese diabetic should be to manage blood sugars with no medication at all. To do that you will have to lose weight. By taking oral medication for control of blood sugar, the diabetic reduces the risk of kidney and eye diseases. Unfortunately, the leading cause of death among diabetics is cardiovascular disease (the increased risk is brought on by diabetes, whether you are thin or fat), and simply controlling blood sugars with oral agents or insulin does not decrease the diabetic's risk of cardiovascular disease.

I have actually had overweight patients who had been counseled to eat more when their blood sugar levels dropped to very low levels. It is somewhat of a chicken-and-egg concept. Which should happen first? Should the doctor lower the patient's medication, or should the patient try to follow a better diet? If your blood sugar levels are high, you will need to follow a better diet before your doctor can lower your medication dosages. If your blood sugar levels are already well maintained, you are eating a diet relatively high in starch, and you are overweight, ask your doctor about starting a better diet and simultaneously cutting back some of your medication.

One of my own success stories is a patient who was significantly overweight, taking 100 units of insulin twice a day, with relatively poor blood sugar control. After I explained the concepts of his illness to him and worked with his diet, he ultimately lost 65 pounds and now uses 30 units or less of insulin twice daily. His blood sugar levels are near normal. I am not sure whether this patient will be able to completely escape the use of medication or insulin, but his insulin therapy is markedly lowered and his blood sugar levels are much better controlled.

I ask my diabetic patients to follow my three basic rules. I do believe that the diabetic diet has too much starch and/or carbohydrate in it for patients who are gaining weight on that diet. There is one positive aspect of the diabetic diet—it teaches the concept of carbohydrate substitution. I ask my diabetic patients to eat no more than one slice of bread or its equivalent with breakfast and lunch. The rule of *No White at Night* still applies, and diabetics can consume all the salad and nonstarchy vegetables they choose at night. It is especially important for diabetics to avoid sugary fruits that raise blood sugar levels quickly, such as oranges, grapes, and raisins. People with diabetes should especially strive to follow a diet that favors low-glycemic-index and low-glycemic-load foods (see Table 6, page 46). Those foods will cause fewer glucose spikes and should require less insulin to maintain normal blood sugars.

An exercise program is important for anyone who wants to lose weight and is especially important for diabetics. Exercise helps drive blood sugar levels down by driving the blood sugar into the muscle groups. Developing an exercise program such as walking will help lower your blood sugar levels and decrease your need for insulin or medication. Combining an exercise program with a change in your diet will only speed the process of losing weight.

As I noted earlier in this chapter, my mother has a personal history of diabetes. She has a strong family history of diabetes, and, as with many diabetics, this has become more of an issue as she has gotten older. Finally, she began gaining weight as her doctor put her on medications to control her blood sugar. With the medication she progressively became heavier with only marginal control of her blood sugars.

My mother became more and more frustrated and finally asked about some of the successes of my own patients using the Three-Rule Diet. My mother's goal was to lose weight to get off her diabetic medication. She started a daily walking program and tries to walk twice daily, if possible. She started her version of *No White at Night* with "no white at lunch" as well. Ultimately, when her weight loss seemed to plateau after several months, she went to "no white at all." She essentially cut all starch out of her diet but continued to eat unlimited amounts of salad and nonstarchy vegetables. She also favored fruits in the morning that had a low glycemic load (see Table 6, page 46). That is the level of starch restriction it took for my mother to achieve progressive weight loss.

Rather than feel deprived by the changes she has had to

make in her diet, she could not be happier. My mother's weight is down 35 pounds. She is no longer taking any medications for her diabetes, and her blood sugars are actually better controlled than they were when she was taking medications but weighed significantly more. Finally, people are telling her she looks great and have been asking her how to lose weight. For my mother, life does not get any better than that.

Diabetes is an illness often caused by obesity in adults. If you can treat your obesity, you can often markedly improve or possibly even eradicate your diabetes. Losing weight is more difficult for diabetics if they are on medication. Weight loss becomes a balancing act between exercise, diet, and a gradual reduction in your diabetes medication. The most important person in that balancing act is you. When you change your exercise pattern and diet you will have better control of your blood sugar and make it easier for your physician to reduce your diabetes medicine. You will probably find it relatively slow going at first, but as your diabetes medicine levels go down, your weight loss will get easier. Almost uniformly when patients stop their diabetes medications and are following a good diet and exercise program, their weight loss will accelerate.

SO, DOC, WHAT SHOULD I EAT?

NOW THAT YOU'VE HEARD the three rules, you should start to think about how you are going to apply them. This means finding foods you like that meet the criteria of the three rules. As you go through this chapter, write down what you eat now at each meal and analyze it. Does what you eat now fit with the three rules (three meals a day, protein at every meal, and no white at night)? If not, think about how you can modify what you are eating. As you read this chapter, write down some reasonable options for each meal.

You will need to learn more about what you are eating. With the nutrition facts printed on most food packages, it is not difficult to understand the breakdown of that food group. I would like to review some basics of food label reading with you. The label will tell you the *total* number of calories. It will also tell you the components of the food, such as fat, carbohydrate, and protein. Unfortunately, the components are not given as a percentage of total calories, so you cannot readily apply the concept of the 40-30-30 balance without doing some simple math. The absolute amounts of protein, fat, and carbohydrate are given by weight in grams, and that is useful. If you intend to use a given food group as a protein source, make sure that it has adequate protein. Any meal should have a minimum of 10 to 20 grams of protein.

It is important to remember that you will be combining some foods to make a meal. Let's use the example of nonfat yogurt and string cheese. The yogurt has 110 calories with no fat. The yogurt has 20 grams of carbohydrate and 7 grams of protein per serving. The string cheese has 80 calories per stick and contains 6 grams of fat and 7 grams of protein per serving. The combination of yogurt and two sticks of string cheese is an overall excellent meal and reasonably balanced. The combination produces 20 grams of carbohydrate, 21 grams of protein, and 12 grams of fat.

I arrived at this combination with some experimentation over time and did not really check the exact content of the food groups until after I had been eating this for lunch for at least six months. Although the exact percentages are not 40-30-30, they are close enough. The 40-30-30 percentages are a good target, but we can certainly vary that meal to meal. Use the nutritional facts in labels to give you some general guidelines. Then, check the numbers more closely on specific food groups that you really like. If you are doing well with your weight-loss program, don't sweat the small stuff. If you are struggling with your weight loss, you need to pay attention to the details.

I would propose some general guidelines that you can consider when you look at the absolute number of grams of the various food groups. Remember that you are trying to target a 40-30-30 balance. It does *not* have to be exact.

The important point is whether this meal satisfies your hunger and keeps you from getting hungry for an additional four to five hours. Add up the various categories of carbohydrate, protein, and fat from the various food serving groups that you are eating. A good rule of thumb is that every meal should have at least 10 to 20 grams of carbohydrate. The amount of protein in grams should be slightly higher but no lower than three-fourths the amount of carbohydrate. Remember, protein has only 4 calories per gram versus 5 calories for carbohydrate. Finally, the amount of fat should be roughly half the amount of carbohydrate. These simple proportions will allow you to come close to the 40-30-30 rules for any given snack or meal.

One of my goals in developing the rules for the *No White at Night* program was to help people avoid tedious calculations. I would like to tell you that there is a very simple way to avoid having to do any calculations. If you strongly favor salads and vegetables as your carbohydrate sources at lunch and dinner, you can probably forgo any calculations. You will simply need to make sure that you have an adequate low-fat protein source. By favoring salads and vegetables you will be dramatically lowering the energy density in the foods you eat. By making that simple change in your carbohydrate intake you will almost certainly cut out several hundred calories per meal and also increase the amount of fiber, vitamins, and other macronutrients in your diet. You will also be moving your diet back toward the foodstuffs that we were all genetically designed to eat.

Usually the hardest part of the diet is finding the lean protein sources (see the list on page 38) you like, so let's start with breakfast. People usually eat some type of starch with breakfast. It may be toast, an English muffin, or oatmeal. I would favor the oatmeal or some type of nonwhite, whole-grain bread. Good breakfast protein sources are Canadian bacon, egg whites, peanut butter, soynut butter if you are allergic to peanut butter, smoked salmon, and turkey bacon. An excellent simple breakfast choice is peanut butter on a piece of whole-wheat toast. Many of my patients do not eat breakfast, but remember, the first rule of the *No White at Night* diet is three meals a day. For breakfast-impaired individuals, I advise peanut butter on a piece of nonwhite toast. It is simple, and it is very balanced so you will not get hungry until lunchtime. If you are time constrained in the morning, try peanut butter on an toasted English muffin. If you choose some type of processed meat such as ground turkey sausage, be sure that it has a low fat content. Lean turkey sausage would have 2 to 4 grams of fat per serving. Lox would have a higher fat content of 6 to 7 grams, but it is a "good fat" that is high in essential fatty acids. Simply look at the package and check the component percentages. I said you would not have to use a calculator, but you will have to read labels.

Peanut butter is an excellent foodstuff to show the importance of reading labels. Many people are concerned about the oils in peanut butter and buy the reduced-fat brands. Unfortunately, most peanut butter manufacturers replace the oil they remove with added sugar. Reduced-fat peanut butter often has as many calories as the regular variety, or more. I recommend that you buy your favorite regular brand of peanut butter, creamy or crunchy.

I also propose that you try to find a 100 percent natural peanut butter. Although peanut butter does have a significant amount of fat, the fats in it are monounsaturated or polyunsaturated and can actually raise your good cholesterol and lower your bad cholesterol. Most commercial peanut butter varieties simply bubble hydrogen through natural peanut butter, which negates some of the advantage of this natural fat. Some of my patients shop at stores where they will actually grind the peanuts for you. A common variety of natural peanut butter is the Adams brand. The brand favored in the Gavin household is Maranatha. Check with your local grocer and see what varieties may be available to you. If you are allergic to peanuts, consider almond or soy butter. They are just as beneficial.

I would like to make some special points about eggs. Eggs are often maligned in the public press. Egg whites are a wonderful balanced source of protein. You can literally live on egg whites as your only source of protein. They are also a relatively inexpensive source of protein. An egg yolk is a 200-mg cholesterol pill. All the protein in the egg is in the whites, and all the cholesterol is in the yolks. If you like eggs, consider having three in the morning but only one yolk per day. If you have a medical condition that mandates a very reduced cholesterol intake, try the egg whites alone. For those who do not want to hassle with separating eggs, consider Egg Beaters.

I eat three hard-boiled egg whites per day during the week. I make egg-white omelets on the weekend when I have more time. You can really make the omelets flavorful with salsa, green onions, or vegetables. If you want to add some cheese, try mozzarella. You can also add lean meat like Canadian bacon. I used to give our dog all the egg yolks until a veterinarian friend told me I would kill the dog, so now he only gets one. Dogs use cholesterol for making the oils in their coat and they love the taste, but remember, the limit is one per day.

You should try to get at least 10 to 20 grams of protein at your breakfast meal. Your breakfast protein will help keep you from being hungry until lunchtime. The worst breakfast choice that you could make is not to eat breakfast at all. By skipping a meal you are only increasing your likelihood of overeating later. You need to eat breakfast even if you are not hungry. If you have a significant time constraint in the morning, consider again a piece of toast or an English muffin with peanut butter. It is quick and easy. If even that is too much of a time delay, consider using something like Carnation Instant Breakfast, Slim-Fast, or some type of breakfast bar that has a balance between the food groups of carbohydrate, protein, and fat in the range of 40-30-30. Breakfast is your most important meal. Do not skip it, even if you are not hungry.

Lunch is a little more straightforward. Most people already know what type of protein sources they like. Excellent protein sources include lean lunchmeat, tuna fish, low-fat cottage cheese, nonfat yogurt, and string cheese. As I said before, this is not about what I like; this is about what you like. If you eat sandwiches, think about using just one slice of bread. Use the same amount of protein or meat but just have half the bread. Another option is to toast the bread and build your sandwich with the outer leaves of a head of lettuce providing the upper layer.

An excellent lunch for people on the run is nonfat yogurt and string cheese. The nonfat yogurt can be flavored with fruit; it does not have to be plain. I realize that not all people like yogurt, but if you do, I strongly recommend that you try this. When you buy yogurt, make sure you read how much protein your favorite brand has. A co-worker in my office pointed out the wide variance in protein content between the different types of nonfat yogurt.

By reading labels and getting advice from friends and co-workers, I have found that the types of yogurt available are actually fairly complicated. Yogurt now comes in several varieties including regular, low-fat, and nonfat. Not only does the amount of fat content decrease as one goes to the non-fat variety, but the amount of sugar also drops as well. There is, however, a marked variation in the amount of protein versus sugar that makes up the average 110 calories in a serving of fruit-flavored nonfat yogurt. In our local area, the yogurts with the highest protein and the lowest sugar content are Albertson's nonfat store brand and Fred Meyer's nonfat store brand. Ironically, they are also some of the least expensive. Yogurt manufacturers vary significantly by region, and I strongly encourage you to read the labels of your local varieties and choose those that have the highest protein and the lowest sugar.

The variability of the different yogurts is a good example of why it is important to read labels. Yoplait fat-free yogurt has 100 calories, with 17 grams of carbohydrate and 5 grams of protein. Lucerne fat-free yogurt has 180 calories, with 33 grams of carbohydrate and 11 grams of protein. Finally, the Fred Meyer store-brand Lite has 100 calories, with 17 grams of carbohydrate and 9 grams of protein. As you can see, there is a tremendous range between the number of calories and the protein content of the various yogurt brands. In this example, the Fred Meyer brand is the best, and my standard lunch choice.

In nonfat yogurt there is a marked range in the level of carbohydrate and protein for the same number of calories. I strongly recommend that you find a nonfat yogurt that has about 8 to 10 grams of protein per serving. If you add string cheese to nonfat yogurt, you add protein and fat, which gives a very good blend of carbohydrate, protein, and fat. I favor nonfat yogurt and string cheese for lunch. I have found that by eating this I am usually not hungry for 4 or 5 hours and my energy level is excellent. I strongly recommend this lunch combination to people who are on the go or on the road, such as truck drivers. If you plan ahead, you will not have to make bad choices in fast-food restaurants or convenience stores. Never skip lunch, even if you are not hungry. Skipping lunch, like skipping breakfast, just causes you to overeat later in the day.

Many times people get hungry at 4:00 or 5:00 and need a snack. I strongly recommend that you consider eating some type of snack if your dinner is going to be delayed until 6:00 or 7:00. By eating a balanced food between 4:00 and 5:00 you will not get so hungry that you will make a bad food choice at 6:00 or 7:00. I keep a box of Balance bars that are designed along the 40-30-30 blend in my office for those times when I know I am going to be late getting home. Other good snack alternatives include cut-up vegetables such as carrots and celery, celery and peanut butter, string cheese, low-fat cheddar, Monterey Jack, peanuts, or fruit such as bananas, pears, or apples. Bad choices for snacking include sugar-based foods such as cookies, candy, or carbonated soft drinks with sugar.

Remember to drink large amounts of water throughout the day. If you have had a previous habit of drinking numerous cans of a regular carbonated soft drink such as Coca-Cola or Pepsi throughout the day, stop it. The bad news is that those cans of soft drink each has 240 calories of sugar. The good news is that if you have been drinking that many cans of soda throughout the day, just stopping that alone will make a huge difference in your ability to lose weight. People who have consumed at least a six-pack of a soft drink throughout the day usually will lose a large amount of weight, on the order of 20 pounds in two months, as their sugar intake dramatically falls.

I favor any type of water-based drink, including water with lemon or lime, iced tea, Crystal Light, and any of the sugar-free soft drinks. Medical researchers have theorized that diet colas such as Diet Coke, Diet Pepsi, and Diet RC have some insulin-like properties. I used to consume Diet Coke or Diet Pepsi at lunch, but changed after reading those reports. I think if you want to optimize your chances of weight loss you should consider doing the same. Good choices are water and any of the noncola diet soft drinks.

Dinner is probably the easiest meal at which to apply the principles. You can have a reasonable portion of whatever lean protein source you like. It may be meat, fish, or fowl. A common visual reference would be a piece of fowl the size of a standard chicken breast. You could also consider a piece of meat the size of the palm of your hand or at least the size of a package of cigarettes. As a cardiologist, I recommend that you think in terms of the size of the palm of your hand. Cooking techniques such as broiling and barbecuing are best, and a number of my patients use the cooking style made popular by the George Foreman grill, which drains away the fat as you cook.

Remember, you can have all the salad and nonstarchy vegetables you want. Experiment with different salad dressings and different types of vinegar to find combinations you like. Try to use the lowest-fat-content salad dressings that taste good to you and use them in moderation. As I said before, this is about finding foods you like and can enjoy eating over the long term. It may take some time, but I am sure you will be fascinated with how you come to appreciate foods that you had not thought about before.

Dessert is a real problem if you are actively trying to lose weight. Remember, to achieve weight loss you need to achieve a calorie deficit. Most desserts, especially in restaurants, are high in refined sugar and fat. I have never understood why we would serve something that is high in sugar so late in the day. There may be special occasions when you are visiting a friend's house and they have prepared some special pie or cake. Consider taking a slice of the dessert home and having it for breakfast the next morning. I love apple pie, and whenever someone makes one and serves it at a dinner I am attending, I ask if I can bring home a slice for breakfast the next day. I do not eat it as dessert. In place of dessert, consider having some fruit such as an apple or pear. Also, consider having a small piece of low-fat cheese.

There are times that you may want a special treat. I encourage you to have it at the end of your meal. A small piece of dark chocolate is an excellent example. By eating the chocolate when you are already "full" you will eat much less of it. In addition, the other foods in your meal will slow the absorption of the sugar in the chocolate, thus lowering its glycemic index. The total calories, however, are still important. For that reason, have as small a piece as you can to quench that urge. And make sure it is dark chocolate, not milk chocolate.

I would like to make a special point about alcohol. Alcohol has a significant number of calories. The calories are entirely carbohydrate in nature. A glass of wine or a bottle of beer can easily be 180 to 240 calories. Some beneficial changes in cholesterol levels are associated with drinking half a glass of red wine per day. If you are interested in optimizing your cholesterol status and choose to drink wine, I suggest that you drink half a glass of red wine after dinner.

Alcohol calories are relatively empty and they do not curb your hunger. By drinking your wine after dinner, you are more likely to enjoy it slowly and feel comfortable limiting yourself to only half a glass. If you have been able to achieve an adequate degree of weight loss and are ready to start adding carbohydrate back into your evening meal, consider adding your carbohydrate as alcohol. A glass or two of wine or one or two bottles of beer is equivalent in calories to a baked potato. When I was a child the principle of drinking your carbohydrate calories was espoused in the popular "drinking man's diet."

I would like to offer you some simple suggestions for eating at restaurants. If your meal comes with soup or salad, favor the salad. Restaurant soups tend to be high in salt and starch such as rice and potatoes. When your server asks you what type of rice or potatoes you prefer, ask for "double vegetables, no starch please." With the popularity of very-low-carbohydrate diets such as the Atkins diet, this is a common request. I have been following this approach for four years now and have never had a restaurant refuse that request or charge me more for it. Finally, you can ask your server not to bring the bread to the table. It is much easier not to eat something if it is not sitting in front of you.

On special occasions when you are out at a restaurant and want to try dessert, order one for the whole table. When I dine out with a group of friends, everyone looks at me, especially when the dessert tray is brought to the table. Usually everyone will pass on ordering a dessert, but when the offer finally comes to me I order the one I think most people will enjoy "with six spoons." It always seems to disappear. Another good option is to select a fruit-and-cheese plate that can be shared among everyone at the table.

Table 8 (see page 82) shows the foods I ate before I changed my diet, the foods I ate while I was actively dieting, and the foods I eat now, while I am maintaining my weight. As I said, it is in part a discovery process. There are foods I eat now that I never ate before. An excellent example is string cheese. My kids actually ate string cheese, but I had never tried it. One day a friend who understood the principles of the Zone diet mentioned to me what a great complement it was to yogurt. I found it interesting because I had been eating yogurt and a banana for lunch and found it very poor in curbing my hunger over a number of hours. When I added a piece of string cheese, my hunger was markedly reduced. I then got rid of the banana and added a second stick of string cheese and that was ideal. Finally, a member of my staff pointed out the differences in protein content between the various nonfat yogurts, and I ultimately arrived at the combination of food that I eat for lunch today. This process evolved over two years.

	TABLE 8 My Diet		
	Overweight	**Dieting**	**Maintenance**
6:00 A.M.	Bagel Jelly	English muffin Jelly Egg whites (3)	English muffin Jelly Egg whites (3) Peanut butter
8:30 A.M.	Pastry	Nothing	Nothing
12:00 noon	Sandwich (½) Veggie sticks	Nonfat yogurt String cheese	Nonfat yogurt String cheese
4:00 P.M.	Snickers bar	Nothing	Balance bar
7:00 P.M.	Meat/fish/fowl Rice Salad or vegetable 1–2 glasses red wine	Meat/fish/fowl Vegetables Salad ½ glass red wine	Meat/fish/fowl Vegetables Salad 1–2 glasses red wine

I am sure you will find different foods in your experiments that ultimately are adopted into your routine meals.

At this point you should have a good idea of what you will eat at breakfast, lunch, and dinner. You may want to write those foods down. If you are still uncertain what you might have with certain meals, see the tables in the appendix. Remember to make food choices you like so that it will be easier to maintain a long-term approach to eating better.

As I look back on my previous diet and consider what I eat now, there are several prominent contrasts. When I had a significant obesity problem, I never ate protein at breakfast. I often ate frequently during the morning because I would get hungry before lunch. I usually ate a fairly reasonable

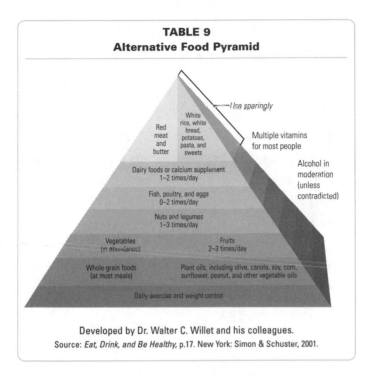

TABLE 9
Alternative Food Pyramid

Use sparingly

Red meat and butter

White rice, white bread, potatoes, pasta, and sweets

Multiple vitamins for most people

Alcohol in moderation (unless contradicted)

Dairy foods or calcium supplement 1–2 times/day

Fish, poultry, and eggs 0–2 times/day

Nuts and legumes 1–3 times/day

Vegetables (in abundance)

Fruits 2–3 times/day

Whole-grain foods (at most meals)

Plant oils, including olive, canola, soy, corn, sunflower, peanut, and other vegetable oils

Daily exercise and weight control

Developed by Dr. Walter C. Willet and his colleagues.
Source: *Eat, Drink, and Be Healthy,* p.17. New York: Simon & Schuster, 2001.

amount of protein at lunch. My afternoon snack is far different and far better at keeping me from getting hungry until dinner. I have given up fruits that have high sugar content or are high in what is commonly referred to as the glycemic index (see Table 6, page 46). Fruits such as oranges, tangerines, and grapes raise your blood sugar level quickly, and then it drops just as quickly. I have given up orange juice and other high-sugar drinks. Finally, I eat considerably more vegetables than I ever did before. In summary, I eat more vegetables, I eat less starch, and I make sure I eat some lean protein early in the day. I think all of these are good changes to anyone's diet. I know these changes have worked for me.

As I stated earlier in the book, I believe that the current USDA Food Guide Pyramid (see Table 5, page 32) promotes eating excess starches and carbohydrate. Other alternative food pyramids have been published. I propose that you follow the food pyramid promoted by Dr. Walter Willett in his book *Eat, Drink, and Be Healthy* (see Table 9, page 83). Dr. Willett relegates the starches to the very top of the pyramid. The bottom of the pyramid is actually daily exercise and weight control. If you follow the principles of *No White at Night* and increase your intake of whole grains, vegetables, and fruits, this should be relatively straightforward. Remember, you are not simply trying to lose weight. This is an opportunity to learn to eat better for a lifetime.

10

DOC, THIS IS NOT WORKING

OST PEOPLE WHO READ this book and follow its principles will be able to achieve weight loss. Some people fail to lose weight, however, and I have come to recognize certain patterns. Men and women, I believe, fail my diet for different reasons. So, I am going to deal first with the issue of men who fail to lose weight, and then women.

The primary reason men fail to lose weight on my diet is that they simply are not following it. I can honestly say that I have never known a male patient or friend who followed the *No White at Night* principles and did not lose weight. Men have more muscle mass and a higher metabolic rate than women do. On average, men can tolerate a higher carbohydrate intake then women can. A major problem with men is usually motivation. Their spouse may think the diet is a great idea and may be preparing appropriate meals at home. When I counsel my male patients regarding the diet and its principles, I often ask, "Who does the cooking at home?" Commonly it is the wife, and she usually will listen intently. What she cannot control is what her husband may eat outside the home, or if he simply refuses to follow the three rules. No dietary program will work for anyone not motivated to follow it.

When I was a kid, my parents struggled with how to help me lose weight until one day in seventh grade I decided I was fat. I then went on a weight-loss program I designed with my mother and returned to a normal body size. My parents were concerned and loving, but no dietary program they proposed was going to work until I decided that I needed to lose weight. It is no different for my patients. Nothing can replace motivation.

A second reason why men fail in the Three-Rule Diet is that they simply do not understand their food groups. When a patient fails to lose weight, I often ask what they eat for breakfast, lunch, and dinner. Not uncommonly, a male patient will tell me he eats cereal, orange juice, and a banana for breakfast. I listen intently and then ask him, "Where's the protein in this breakfast?" He thinks about it for a few seconds and then softly responds, "The cereal?" My male patients have a much poorer understanding of the makeup of their foods than my female patients. These men often respond to additional education. If you think you are in this category, consider visiting a dietitian who will work with you on the principles of the Three-Rule Diet.

It has been my experience in counseling patients through my office that the principles of *No White at Night* routinely work for men. If you have limited physical activity due to some type of medical problem, or you wish to increase your rate of weight loss, you may also consider using the principles of *No White at Night* as described shortly. If you are male and struggling with insufficient weight loss, then I recommend that you maintain a food diary for several days and seek the counsel of a dietitian in your area to ensure that you are not getting excess calories in your diet from a source that you do not recognize.

My female patients tend to be more motivated and have a better understanding of the various food groups. Women start with the disadvantage of a slower rate of metabolism than men and may also have something in their genetic code that makes them less able to give up stored fat calories. Women probably on average have a greater tendency to gain weight more than men at any given carbohydrate level in their diet. Whereas the average male can probably consume a 50 percent carbohydrate diet, the average female is more likely to consume on the order of 40 percent. That means that some women may need to achieve as low as 20 to 30 percent carbohydrate intake before they can lose weight. My mother is an excellent example of this concept. Her weight loss stalled with "no white at lunch," and she ultimately achieved long-term success by going to "no white at all."

Motivated people having difficulty will have to do more

pencil work by keeping a food diary. Write down, for at least two or three days, everything that you eat. Then analyze those foods for their calories and various components of carbohydrate, protein, and fat. Once you have established what you are eating and that the proportions are right, consider further reducing the amount of carbohydrate in your diet. The goal is to take your carbohydrate level from roughly 40 percent down to 30 percent. Try getting rid of or markedly reducing your carbohydrate intake at lunch. You can still have unlimited salad and vegetables. Apply the *No White at Night* rule to lunch. If that still is not adequate, try getting rid of your starch intake at breakfast as well. When you incorporate these changes, you are moving your carbohydrate intake as a percentage of your total calories closer to that of the Atkins diet. By following the other principles, however, you will not increase your fat intake on an absolute basis. Also, in contrast to the Atkins diet, you are still allowed to have unlimited salad and nonstarchy vegetables.

You will be moving your personal diet percentages toward the left side of Table 4 (see page 24) in the diet spectrum. By following the other principles, however, you will not increase your fat intake on an absolute basis. Also, in contrast to the Atkins diet, you are still allowed to have unlimited salad and nonstarchy vegetables.

Table 10 (see page 89) shows you a simple algorithm for intensifying the *No White at Night* approach. Everyone should be able to start with the simple principles of *No White at Night*. If you believe that starches are a major cause of your obesity problem and suspect that you may be one of

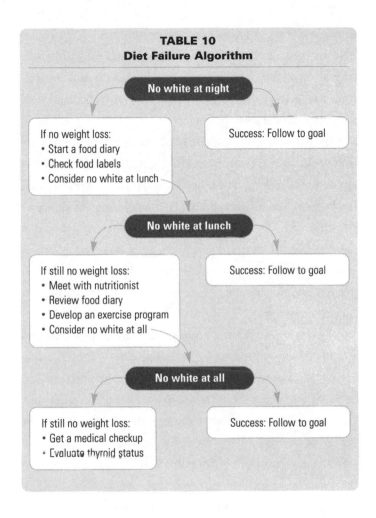

TABLE 10
Diet Failure Algorithm

No white at night

If no weight loss:
• Start a food diary
• Check food labels
• Consider no white at lunch

Success: Follow to goal

No white at lunch

If still no weight loss:
• Meet with nutritionist
• Review food diary
• Develop an exercise program
• Consider no white at all

Success: Follow to goal

No white at all

If still no weight loss:
• Get a medical checkup
• Evaluate thyroid status

Success: Follow to goal

those people who can tolerate a carbohydrate intake of only 20 to 30 percent like my mother, you may wish to also start at the "no white at lunch" point. If you achieve short-term success, simply follow the principles of the diet until you reach your target weight. If you are unable to achieve early success, then I recommend that you start a food diary, read labels, and visit a dietitian to review your food diary. If you have any associated medical conditions such as a family history of thyroid problems, or you are taking thyroid medication, I suggest that you consult with your physician and have your medication levels reviewed.

Another important question: If the diet principles are not working for you, have you increased your exercise? Exercise has the benefit of boosting your metabolism and having you expend more calories. Remember, the best way to achieve weight loss over time is a combination of diet and exercise. If you did not start an exercise program, at least consider a walking program. Walking thirty minutes per day should dramatically improve the efficiency of your diet program.

Finally, if you have an adequate exercise program and feel that you have reduced your carbohydrate intake as low as possible, consider seeking professional nutritional advice. Some of my patients have failed to lose weight, even though I have worked with them for more than a year. Over the course of one year I have referred at least six intelligent, motivated women to an intensive nutritional counseling service. It is expensive and it is time-consuming, but each one of these patients has achieved considerable weight loss and has thanked me for referring her to the organization.

I also suggest that you ask your doctor to check your thyroid and see if there is any other reason why you have not been able to lose weight. Most of my patients do not need this type of intensive counseling nor are they willing to put up with the time or expense involved. However, a few individuals have extreme difficulty in losing weight; if following the principles and modifications I have outlined is not working, then I suggest that you take your food diaries and get further counseling.

11

A PAT ON THE BACK

I HAVE COUNSELED hundreds of patients regarding their diet. When I am actively following my patients and trying to help them lose weight, I often see them once a month. When those patients achieve success, which can be losing 2, 4, or even 10 pounds in a month, they often return and feel elated. If you achieve success with these dietary guidelines, and many do, I am sorry that I am not going to be able to share in your happiness.

When patients leave the exam room from their follow-up appointments and have been able to achieve weight loss, I usually congratulate them in front of my nursing staff. My nursing staff, some of whom have also followed the diet with success, share in their happiness as well and congratulate them. Since I am not able to do this in person, I would greatly appreciate it if you would stand in front of a mirror at the end of every month you lose weight, look yourself right in the eye, and say, "Great job." Losing weight is not that hard once you understand the principles. It does, however, take motivation and commitment over time. Now you are fitting into the clothes you have not worn to work in a long time, feeling more energetic, and having friends ask you, "How'd you do it?"

We give my diabetic patients who achieve weight loss the same kudos in the office. The diabetic patients who are able to stop their medications because of weight loss get a special recognition—they get a hug in front of all my staff. Those people, men and women, have dramatically reduced their risk of cardiovascular disease and have overcome the additional hurdle of medications that can contribute to weight gain. That is a real accomplishment.

So I regret that I will not be there to share in your joy, but your friends will be. Many of them will ask how you lost your weight, and you can explain the principles to them as well. Be an example of how motivation, exercise, and diet can cure obesity.

APPENDIX
Recipes

Introduction

THE BEAUTY OF the diet principles in *No White at Night* is that you can adapt them to almost any style of cooking. These recipes are not meant to be an all-inclusive list of foods for you to eat. Rather, they will provide you with some practical examples of how to apply the principles of this book to everyday food. It is important for you to look at the various food groups in every meal you eat. Then ask yourself these basic questions: Is there any protein in this meal? How much carbohydrate is in this meal? Then modify what you are eating so that it meets the guidelines of the three rules.

I want to stress the importance of eating foods that you

enjoy. No long-term change in your eating habits can be successful if you do not enjoy the foods that you are eating or find them interesting. If you do not particularly like eggs at breakfast or you are allergic to peanut butter, that is fine. Simply find another protein source that works for you.

It will be very important for you to read labels of common foods that you eat. You may be very surprised at the high amount of carbohydrate in some foods and the minimal amount of protein. A great example of this is most dry cereals, which are relatively high in sugar and low in protein. I cannot overly stress the importance of reading labels on the foods you most commonly eat.

You start your day with breakfast, and we will start the recipes there, too. You must eat breakfast to have a successful weight-loss program. The worst choice for breakfast is none at all. The next problem I encounter is patients not having any protein in their breakfast. A common example would be the person who chooses to have orange juice, dry cereal, and a banana for breakfast. That type of meal is high in sugar and low in protein. It will lead to a rapid rise and fall in blood sugar and recurrent hunger in several hours.

I would like to propose a simple way to evaluate any meal you eat. If you are hungry an hour or two after eating, you ate inadequate protein at your last meal. If you are sleepy an hour or two after a given meal, then you ate too much carbohydrate at that meal. To combat recurrent hunger, you will need to increase the protein in a meal. To get rid of the drowsiness, you will need to decrease the carbohydrate in a meal. An appropriately balanced meal with adequate protein and carbohydrate should allow you to be alert and free of hunger for at least four hours.

I invite you to go through this recipe section and find foods that you enjoy. The recipes for breakfast and lunch can be interchanged. If you live in a warm climate, you may prefer to have something cool for breakfast such as nonfat yogurt and fruit or cottage cheese and fruit. Some of my patients prefer peanut butter on toast for lunch rather than breakfast. Some of the egg dishes can certainly be eaten throughout the day, including dinner. It is important that if you move a recipe to your evening meal that it follow the *No White at Night* rule. Remember, this is about food that you enjoy and find interesting.

Breakfast

POOR BREAKFAST CHOICES

Worst	No breakfast at all
Bad	No protein with breakfast
Poor	French toast/pancakes/several slices of toast/ pastries/doughnuts/waffles/fruit juice/ most dry cereals

These poor choices are high in refined sugar and have minimal protein, which leads to a rapid rise and fall in your blood sugar and poor control of your hunger.

Protein Boosters					
	Calories	Carbs (g)	Protein (g)	Fat (g)	Saturated Fat (g)
Protein powder	90	2	17.5	1.5	0
Soy protein powder	80	3	14	1	0.5
2 egg whites	34	0	7	0	0
1 oz peanuts	180	5	7	15	0
1 oz almonds	164	6	6	14.5	0
2 slices Canadian bacon	90	1.5	15	3	1
3 oz roasted chicken	75	0	21	1	0
1.5 oz lox or smoked fish	25	3	2	1	1
½ cup skim milk	45	9	4	0	0

RECIPES

English Muffin with Peanut Butter

1 English muffin
2 Tbsp natural peanut butter

✺ Natural peanut butter is the best. Common brands would be Adam's or Maranatha; we find Maranatha easier to spread. Your local grocery store may have its own brand, or even allow you to grind your own. Most of the common brands have altered the fats (partially hydrogenated) to make the peanut butter easier to spread. The natural peanut butter is better for you and will raise your good cholesterol (HDL). Avoid the reduced-fat brands, which have up to three times the sugar of regular. Creamy or crunchy makes no difference. Almond butter and soynut butter are also excellent choices.

> CALORIES: 310   CARBS: 32 G
> PROTEIN: 13 G   FAT: 16 G   SAT. FAT: 2.5 G

Zita's Egg-White Omelet

3 egg whites
1 egg yolk (optional; omit if you are on a low-cholesterol diet)
1 tsp olive oil or cooking spray
diced red or green peppers, chopped green onions, or any
*   vegetables you enjoy*
salt and pepper to taste
½ cup nonfat mozzarella cheese
fresh salsa for garnish (see page 101)

✴ Whisk the egg whites and yolk. Preheat a small skillet and add olive oil or cooking spray. Place mixture in pan and cook over medium heat for 2–4 minutes, covered. Top the egg mixture with the vegetables, salt and pepper to taste, and mozzarella. Cover and cook another 2–4 minutes until done. Serve with salsa.

CALORIES: 369   CARBS: 14 G   PROTEIN: 51.5 G
FAT: 5 G   SAT. FAT: 1.5 G WITH YOLK

Fresh Salsa

1 cup diced plum tomatoes
2 Tbsp chopped green chilies
1 Tbsp minced red onion
1 Tbsp chopped fresh cilantro
1 tsp fresh lime juice
4 cloves garlic, minced
¼ tsp salt
¼ tsp freshly ground black pepper

☀ Combine all ingredients in a small bowl. You can use on eggs, fish, or tortillas. For a bean dip, add 1 cup salsa to 1 can mashed pinto beans.

CALORIES PER ¼-CUP SERVING: 10   CARBS: 2 G
PROTEIN: 0.5 G   FAT: 0 G   SAT. FAT: 0 G

Oatmeal

> ½ cup oatmeal
> 2 Tbsp nonfat milk
> peanuts or almonds (optional)

✸ Cook oatmeal according to instructions on package.

✸ Oatmeal is an excellent breakfast starch. Unfortunately it does not have an adequate amount of protein (less than 5 g). Consider supplementing the oatmeal with one of the protein boosters shown on page 98. You can also add peanuts or almonds to the oatmeal if you choose.

CALORIES: 153   CARBS: 27 G
PROTEIN: 7 G   FAT: O G   SAT. FAT: O G

Canadian Bacon and Eggs

> 2 slices Canadian bacon
> olive oil or cooking spray
> 3 egg whites
> 1 egg yolk (optional)

✸ Place the Canadian bacon on a paper towel and heat in the microwave for 60 seconds. This will reduce the fat. Preheat a medium skillet coated with olive oil or cooking spray over medium heat. Add the bacon and eggs and cook to desired consistency.

CALORIES: 196   CARBS: 1 G   PROTEIN: 25 G
FAT: 10 G   SAT. FAT: 1.5 G

Dry Cereal

1 cup cereal (I recommend Kashi Go Lean)
½ cup nonfat milk

✳ Most dry cereals are high in sugar/carbohydrate and low in protein (usually 2 g or less per serving). You need to read the labels. Make sure you get adequate protein if you eat dry cereal. Even if you do not care for the Kashi brand, consider the contents, especially protein, to be the standard for comparing brands.

CALORIES: 235   CARBS: 39 G
PROTEIN: 13 G   FAT: 3 G   SAT. FAT: 3 G

Linnea's Fruit Smoothie

½ cup nonfat yogurt
½ ripe banana
½ cup strawberries (fresh or frozen) or other fruit
1 cup ice cubes (optional)
1 Tbsp lime juice (optional)
1 scoop soy protein powder

❋ Place all ingredients in a blender and blend until smooth. The banana will produce a creamy texture. The ice cubes and lime juice will thin the smoothie and are optional. You might use frozen fruit rather than ice cubes. A protein supplement or additional protein is needed to make this a complete meal. See the protein boosters shown on page 98.

CALORIES: 238   CARBS: 30 G
PROTEIN: 31 G   FAT: 1 G   SAT. FAT: 0 G

Breakfast Burrito

1 tsp olive oil
½ cup diced onion
¼ cup sliced mushrooms
2 tsp diced green Anaheim chilies
⅓ cup chopped spinach
1 Tbsp diced tomatoes
4 egg whites
2 egg yolks
2 low-carb tortillas
salsa for garnish
cilantro sprigs for garnish

✳ Heat a skillet over medium heat with olive oil. Sauté the onion until soft. Add the mushrooms and chilies and cook until almost dry. Add the spinach and tomatoes and cook until heated through. Set aside. In a separate skillet scramble and cook the eggs until desired consistency. Fold the scrambled eggs into the vegetable mixture. Cook the tortillas in the microwave according to the package instructions. Place the tortillas on plates and divide the egg/vegetable mixture between both. Fold each tortilla over the mixture and garnish with salsa and cilantro sprigs.

CALORIES PER SERVING: 177   CARBS: 6.5 G
PROTEIN: 15 G   FAT: 10 G   SAT. FAT: 1.5 G

Vegetable Frittata

4 egg whites
2 egg yolks
1 Tbsp olive oil
1 medium onion, chopped
¾ cup chopped green, red, or orange peppers
¼ cup chopped Anaheim green chilies
1 Tbsp grated Parmesan cheese
parsley, chopped, for garnish
salt and pepper to taste

✳ Preheat oven to 350 degrees. Beat the eggs in a bowl. Heat the olive oil in a medium ovenproof skillet over medium heat, then add the onion and sauté until brown and beginning to get crispy. Add the peppers and chilies and sauté 1 minute longer. Add the eggs, sprinkle with the Parmesan cheese, and put the pan in the oven. Bake approximately 10 minutes. Garnish with chopped parsley. Add salt and pepper to taste.

CALORIES PER SERVING: 179   CARBS: 9 G
PROTEIN: 6.5 G   FAT: 8 G   SAT. FAT: O G

Potato and Swiss Chard Frittata

2 cups chopped potatoes
1 cup chopped Swiss chard
⅓ cup nonfat milk
3 Tbsp grated Parmesan cheese
2 whole eggs
5 egg whites
salt and pepper to taste
1 tsp butter
⅓ cup grated low-fat mozzarella cheese
Swiss chard slices for garnish (optional)

✳ Preheat broiler. Place potatoes in a medium saucepan, cover with water, and bring to a boil. Reduce heat and simmer about 8 minutes. Add the Swiss chard and continue cooking until tender, then drain. Combine the milk, Parmesan cheese, eggs, and salt and pepper to taste in a large bowl and whisk together. Stir in the potato mixture. Melt the butter in a medium nonstick ovenproof skillet. Pour the egg and potato mixture into the skillet and cook 15 minutes or until the top is just set. Remove from heat and sprinkle with the mozzarella cheese. Broil about 5 minutes or until golden brown. Garnish with Swiss chard slices if desired. Because of the potatoes, this is usually a breakfast or lunch dish.

CALORIES PER SERVING: 188   CARBS: 12.1 G
PROTEIN: 14.7 G   FAT: 8.8 G   SAT. FAT: 3.8 G

Lunch

Lunch is usually an easier meal for people to apply the three rules. Most people eat lunch, and most people eat some protein at lunch. I would like to stress that you should try to find a lean protein source. It is certainly more reasonable to have a turkey sandwich than a bologna sandwich. Unlimited salad and nonstarchy vegetables are acceptable. It then becomes important to limit your additional carbohydrate intake. If you prefer a sandwich for lunch, try to use only one slice of bread. You can have a half sandwich with the usual amount of meat or protein you would normally have on a whole sandwich. Or consider toasting the bottom piece of bread and using an outer leaf of iceberg lettuce as the upper piece of bread for your sandwich. Finally, instead of using bread, substitute a low-carbohydrate tortilla. Make a wrap sandwich with your favorite deli meats and avoid the bread entirely.

The important point is to limit the additional carbohydrate that you may have been eating. Instead of a bag of chips with lunch, pack a bag of carrots and celery. Instead of cookies for dessert, pack an apple. Definitely try to avoid energy-dense foods as accompaniments to your lunch. If lunch is a problem because you are time-pressed, plan something easy. Nonfat yogurt and two pieces of string cheese is very convenient and also very satisfying in relieving your hunger. Nonfat cottage cheese and tomatoes could be another excellent lunch option. When my mother goes to a luncheon where she does not know what is going to be served, she always eats two pieces of string cheese before she walks in the door. That way, in a worst-case scenario, she can simply eat the salad and she will have had a relatively balanced meal. The important point about lunch is to make sure you eat it. You then have to plan on having the right choices. Remember, failing to plan is planning to fail.

Bread Equivalents				
	Serving size	Calories	Carbohydrates	Protein
Bread, white	1 slice	80	18	2
Bread, rye	1 slice	73.5	14	2.5
Bread, whole-wheat	1 slice	74	13	3
Bread, whole-grain	1 slice	50	7	5
English muffin	1	140	27	5
Bagel	1	150	30	6
Tortilla	1 6-inch	159	27	4
Low-carb tortilla	1 6-inch	50	11	5
Bran muffin	1 2.5-oz	190	30	3
Potato, white	1	178.5	41.1	4.2
Rice, white	1 cup	205	45	4
Rice, brown	1 cup	220	46	4
Pasta, white	1 cup	213	39.7	3.8
Corn	½ cup	77	17	3

You can have the equivalent of one slice of bread for breakfast and lunch. If you *must* have two slices of bread with a sandwich, use a low-carbohydrate bread product.

Yogurt and String Cheese

8 oz nonfat yogurt
2 pieces string cheese

✳ The amount of protein versus carbohydrate in your brand of yogurt is very important. You want to look for a brand of flavored nonfat yogurt with at least 7–8 grams of protein. Yoplait has relatively high sugar content and inadequate protein.

CALORIES: 244 CARBS: 17 G
PROTEIN: 21 G FAT: 9 G SAT. FAT: 4 G

Cottage Cheese and Tomatoes

½ cup nonfat cottage cheese
1 medium tomato

CALORIES: 103 CARBS: 9 G
PROTEIN: 15 G FAT: 0 G SAT. FAT: 0 G

Cottage Cheese and Fruit

½ cup nonfat cottage cheese with fruit

CALORIES: 103   CARBS: 9 G
PROTEIN: 15 G   FAT: O G   SAT. FAT: O G

Veggie Sticks

carrot sticks or celery sticks

CALORIES: 31   CARBS: 7 G
PROTEIN: 1 G   FAT: O G   SAT. FAT: O G

Deli Sandwich

1 slice bread, preferably whole-wheat
3 oz turkey or any lean meat
lettuce and tomato

✳ Make your sandwich with only one slice of bread. Try toasting the bread. Build your sandwich from the bottom up. Use the outer leaves of some iceberg lettuce as the top slice of bread. If you really must have two slices of bread, try the new low-carbohydrate alternatives. By making a wrap sandwich with a low-carb tortilla you will also reduce the carbs.

CALORIES: 170   CARBS: 18 G
PROTEIN: 20 G   FAT: 1.5–2 G   SAT. FAT: 0 G

Chicken Wrap Sandwich

2 skinless, boneless chicken breasts, pounded to ¼-in thick
2 Tbsp olive oil
salt and pepper to taste
6-oz bag baby spinach
2 cups whole-milk yogurt, drained overnight
4 cloves garlic, minced
4 low-carb tortillas
6 oz mozzarella or Monterey Jack cheese
2 avocados, peeled and sliced
1 Tbsp fresh lemon juice
hot sauce to taste
2 tomatoes, sliced

✳ Brush the chicken with 1 tbsp oil and season with salt and pepper to taste. Grill or broil chicken, cool, and slice thin. In a pan of boiling water, blanch the spinach for 30 seconds. Drain, cool, squeeze dry, and chop. Mix the spinach with the remaining oil and add salt to taste. Stir in the drained yogurt and the garlic. Season again with salt and pepper as needed. Arrange the tortillas on plates and layer the cheese, avocados, and lemon juice. Season with salt and pepper and hot sauce to taste. Layer the tomatoes, spinach, and chicken. Roll tortillas and wrap in plastic. Refrigerate until firm, then microwave or grill until cheese melts.

CALORIES PER SERVING: 490   CARBS: 11 G
PROTEIN: 34 G   FAT: 34.5 G   SAT. FAT: 10 G

Hot Ham & Cheese

1 slice wheat bread
mustard to taste
low-fat mayonnaise to taste
2 slices deli ham
1 slice nonfat mozzarella cheese
tomato or onion slices (optional)

✹ Toast the bread, spread with mustard and low-fat mayonnaise as desired, place deli ham on toast, and top with cheese. You may want to add some tomato or onion slices between the meat and the cheese. Place under the broiler until the cheese melts or heat in the microwave 30–60 seconds. Serve with salad and vegetable sticks.

> CALORIES: 156   CARBS: 20 G
> PROTEIN: 14 G   FAT: 2.2 G   SAT. FAT: 0 G

Mom's Tomato Soup

1 can nonfat evaporated milk
1 14½-oz can diced tomatoes with basil, oregano, and garlic
salt and pepper to taste

✳ Combine all ingredients in a medium saucepan and cook over low to medium heat. Do not overcook or milk will curdle. Serve when warm.

CALORIES PER SERVING: 134   CARBS: 23 G

PROTEIN: 11 G   FAT: 0 G   SAT. FAT: 0 G

Tomato Eggplant Soup

2 medium eggplants
2 Tbsp olive oil
2 medium onions, chopped
6 cloves garlic, chopped
1 6-oz can tomato paste
8 cups chicken stock
1 cup chopped fresh basil
salt and pepper to taste
Parmesan cheese, grated

✳ Cut eggplants in half and coat with a small amount of olive oil. Roast cut side down on cooking sheet under broiler until the skin bubbles, about 10–15 minutes. Peel the eggplant and cut into chunks. Sauté eggplant, onions, and garlic until soft. Combine eggplant mixture with the tomato paste, chicken stock, basil, and salt and pepper to taste. Simmer about 20 minutes, then purée soup in food processor. Return to pot and heat. Serve with grated Parmesan cheese.

CALORIES PER SERVING: 101   CARBS: 9 G
PROTEIN: 3 G   FAT: 6 G   SAT. FAT: 1 G

Quesadilla

olive oil
2 8-in low-carb tortillas
2 oz sliced or grated mozzarella cheese
cilantro, salsa, guacamole, and/or nonfat sour cream for garnish

✳ Preheat a medium skillet coated with olive oil. Place a tortilla in the pan and cook over medium heat. Add cheese and top with the other tortilla. Cook several minutes, then flip to brown other side so the cheese is thoroughly melted. Garnish with cilantro, salsa, guacamole, and/or nonfat sour cream.

✳ You can add any vegetables, peppers, or meat you desire when you add the cheese. If you want mushrooms and onions, sauté them first. You might also want to sauté the vegetables.

CALORIES: 244   CARBS: 8 G
PROTEIN: 24 G   FAT: 13 G   SAT. FAT: 4 G

Shrimp/Crab Louie

½ head iceberg lettuce, chopped
2 green onions, chopped
1 medium tomato, cut into wedges
2 hard-boiled eggs, sliced
½ lb precooked shrimp or crab
lemon wedge for garnish

✳ Divide lettuce between two plates. Sprinkle on the onions, tomato, and eggs. You may choose to omit the egg yolks if cholesterol is an issue. Pile shrimp or crab in the center. Garnish with the lemon wedge.

✳ Optional additions might be red or green pepper slices, asparagus spears, hearts of palm, or olives. Serve with low-fat Thousand Island dressing. Consider adding salsa to the salad dressing to reduce the calories.

CALORIES PER SERVING: 220   CARBS: 5.5 G
PROTEIN: 35.5 G   FAT: 6 G   SAT. FAT: 1.5 G

Scallops and Mushroom Salad

1 lb scallops
¼ cup chopped green onion
1 lb sliced mushrooms
1 lemon
¼ cup olive oil
salt and pepper to taste
parsley, chopped, for garnish
cherry tomatoes for garnish
1 head Bibb lettuce

✳ Poach scallops in water for 4–5 minutes. Drain and chill. Place scallops, onion, and mushrooms in a bowl, squeeze ½ lemon over the top and toss. Beat remaining lemon juice with olive oil, then add salt and pepper to taste. Pour over scallops. Before serving, garnish with parsley and tomatoes. Serve on lettuce leaves.

CALORIES PER SERVING: 249   CARBS: 9 G
PROTEIN: 21.5 G   FAT: 14 G   SAT. FAT: 0 G

Steak Salad

3 cloves garlic, minced

¼ tsp salt

¼ tsp black pepper

1 lb boneless sirloin steak

olive oil or cooking spray

10 cups torn Romaine lettuce

8 slices tomato

4 slices red onion, separate rings

2 Tbsp crumbled blue cheese

½ cup simple balsamic vinaigrette dressing

✳ Combine garlic, salt, and pepper, and rub over both sides of the steak. Place steak on a grill or broiler pan coated with olive oil or cooking spray. Broil 4 minutes on each side or to desired degree of doneness. Divide lettuce among four plates. Lay tomato slices on lettuce and add onion slices over tomato. Slice steak across the grain into ¼-inch-thick slices and add over salad. Sprinkle each serving with blue cheese and drizzle with vinaigrette.

CALORIES PER SERVING: 259   CARBS: 15.8 G
PROTEIN: 29 G   FAT: 8.5 G   SAT. FAT: 3.5 G

Tuna Slaw with Oil and Vinegar

¼ cup thinly sliced sweet onion
6 cups thinly sliced green cabbage
¼ cup canola oil
½ cup cider or white vinegar
1 tsp sugar or sweetener
dash Tabasco sauce
dash salt-free Spike
black pepper to taste
1 6-oz can water-packed albacore tuna, drained

✹ Toss all ingredients except tuna together. Divide between two plates and put tuna on top.

CALORIES PER SERVING: 187   CARBS: 21 G
PROTEIN: 15 G   FAT: 7 G   SAT. FAT: 0 G

Cheryl's Curried Chicken Soup

3 Tbsp butter
1½ Tbsp flour
2 tsp curry powder
4 cups chicken broth or stock
½ large onion, chopped
3 large carrots, grated
1 egg yolk
4 Tbsp light cream
2 cooked chicken breasts, chopped
paprika for garnish
4 green onions, sliced diagonally, for garnish

✳ Make roux with the butter, flour, and curry powder by melting butter in skillet, adding flour slowly, then curry powder. Heat until desired color and thickness are obtained. Whisk in the chicken broth and bring to a boil. Add the onion and carrots and simmer 5 minutes, or until onion is tender. In a bowl whisk together the egg yolk and light cream and slowly add to the soup while stirring. Add the chicken pieces and simmer 10 minutes. Serve in bowls and garnish with paprika and green onions.

CALORIES PER SERVING: 140   CARBS: 9 G
PROTEIN: 15.7 G   FAT: 4.5 G   SAT. FAT: .35 G

Vegetable Soup

SERVES 4

2 Tbsp olive oil

2 large onions, coarsely chopped

3 cloves garlic, crushed

1½ cups sliced carrots

1½ cups sliced celery

⅔ cup sliced mushrooms

1 medium zucchini, sliced

3½ cups chicken broth

1 16-oz can Italian plum tomatoes, undrained

1 tsp crumbled dried oregano

½ tsp crumbled dried basil

⅛ tsp freshly ground black pepper

¼ tsp hot sauce, or to taste

¼–½ tsp salt-free all-purpose seasoning

8 Tbsp Parmesan cheese, freshly grated, for garnish

✻ Add the olive oil to a large skillet over medium-high heat, and sauté onions, garlic, carrots, celery, and mushrooms about 4–5 minutes. Add zucchini and sauté another 4–5 minutes. Add chicken broth and tomatoes and stir. Add oregano, basil, pepper, hot sauce, and seasoning and bring to boil. Reduce heat, cover, and simmer 8–12 minutes, or until vegetables are tender-crisp. Ladle into bowls and top each serving with Parmesan cheese.

CALORIES PER SERVING: 109   CARBS: 10 G
PROTEIN: 6 G   FAT: 6 G   SAT. FAT: 2 G

Shrimp Salad

SALAD:

½ lb cooked, peeled, and deveined medium shrimp

1 cup chopped tomato

¼ cup chopped red onion

½ cup chopped cucumber

1½ tsp minced jalapeno chilies

2 Tbsp minced fresh cilantro

DRESSING:

6 Tbsp nonfat sour cream

⅓ cup reduced-fat cream cheese, softened

1½ Tbsp fresh lime juice

½ tsp sea salt

¼ tsp ground white pepper

lettuce leaves

avocados, tomatoes, and lemon wedges for garnish

❋ Combine all the salad ingredients in a large bowl and refrigerate. Combine all the dressing ingredients in a small bowl and whisk until smooth. Gently stir the dressing into the shrimp mixture. Refrigerate 30 minutes before serving. You can put lettuce cups on each plate and spoon salad into cups. Garnish with avocados, tomatoes, and lemon wedges.

CALORIES PER SERVING: 110   CARBS: 8 G
PROTEIN: 15 G   FAT: 1.5 G   SAT. FAT: 0

Freddy's Special

1 6-oz can water-packed albacore tuna, drained
1 15-oz can cannellini beans or garbanzo beans, drained
2 Tbsp light olive oil
juice of ½ lemon
¼ cup chopped sweet white onion
1 clove garlic, minced
1 Tbsp fresh chopped parsley
freshly ground black pepper to taste

✳ Combine all ingredients in a bowl and chill. Because of the garbanzo beans, this is usually a lunch dish.

CALORIES: 93   CARBS: 8 G
PROTEIN: 5 G   FAT: 4.5 G   SAT. FAT: 0.6 G

Grammy's Gazpacho

1 cup chopped tomato

⅓ cup finely chopped red bell pepper

½ cup finely chopped celery

½ cup finely chopped cucumber

¼ cup diced red onion

¼ cup diced tomatillos

1 tsp extra-virgin olive oil

¼ cup diced carrot

¼ cup diced jicama

1 tsp chopped chives

2–3 Tbsp red wine vinegar

2 Tbsp olive oil

2 cups vegetable juice cocktail or tomato juice

½ tsp Worcestershire sauce

¼ cup chopped fresh cilantro

1 tsp minced garlic

½ tsp sea salt, or to taste

¼ tsp white pepper, or to taste

1 tsp finely chopped jalapeno chilies (optional)

✳ Combine all ingredients, cover, and chill thoroughly.
Taste and adjust the seasoning with additional salt and white
pepper, if desired.

> CALORIES PER SERVING: 72   CARBS: 7 G
> PROTEIN: 1.5 G   FAT: 4 G   SAT. FAT: 0 G

Tuna-Salad Pita Sandwiches

1 hard-boiled egg
1 tsp lemon juice
dash black pepper
1 6-oz tuna steak or 1 6-oz can water-packed tuna, drained
cooking spray
¼ cup diced celery
2 Tbsp minced green onion
3 Tbsp reduced-fat mayonnaise
1 tsp Dijon mustard
¼ cup chopped dill pickle
2 5-in whole-wheat pitas, cut in half
1¼ cups torn Bibb lettuce
4 tomato slices, ¼-in thick

✻ Slice egg in half lengthwise; discard yolk if cholesterol is an issue. Dice egg halves and set aside. Prepare grill or broiler. Sprinkle lemon juice and pepper over tuna. Place tuna on a grill or broiler rack coated with cooking spray. Cook 4 minutes on each side or until tuna is medium-rare or to desired doneness. Coarsely chop tuna. Combine tuna, diced egg, celery, onion, mayonnaise, mustard, and pickle in a bowl. Line each pita half with ⅓ cup lettuce and 2 tomato slices. Divide tuna mixture evenly among pita halves.

CALORIES PER SERVING: 327   CARBS: 19.5 G
PROTEIN: 30 G   FAT: 14.25 G   SAT. FAT: 1.5 G

Favorite Turkey Chili

1 Tbsp cooking oil

1 lb extra-lean ground turkey

1 onion, chopped

1 clove garlic, minced

3 large tomatoes, diced

1 8-oz can tomato sauce

1 Tbsp chili powder

1 Tbsp chopped oregano

4 Tbsp chopped fresh cilantro

½ tsp cumin

½ tsp salt

1 29-oz can red kidney beans, drained

¼ cup nonfat yogurt

✳ Heat oil in 4-quart saucepan. Add turkey and fry until crumbly. Add onion, garlic, tomatoes, tomato sauce, chili powder, oregano, 2 Tbsp cilantro, cumin, and salt. Cover and cook on low 1 hour. Add beans. Cover and heat. Spoon in bowls and top with yogurt and remaining cilantro.

CALORIES PER SERVING: 238   CARBS: 29 G
PROTEIN: 28 G   FAT: 4 G   SAT. FAT: 0 G

Chicken Caesar Salad

SALAD:

1 head Romaine lettuce
2 Roma tomatoes, quartered
4 chicken breast halves, cooked and sliced

VINAIGRETTE:

1 egg
juice of 1 lemon
dash Tabasco sauce
salt and freshly ground black pepper to taste
½ cup extra-virgin olive oil
½ cup grated Parmesan cheese

✳ To prepare salad, tear lettuce into pieces and add tomatoes and chicken. To prepare vinaigrette, coddle the egg by boiling it in a pan of water for 20 seconds. Remove the egg, crack it, and scoop out the inside into a small bowl. Add the lemon juice, Tabasco sauce, and salt and pepper to taste. Whisk until well combined. Add the olive oil in a slow stream as you whisk. Pour over salad, add three-quarters of the cheese, and toss well. Sprinkle with the remainder of the cheese and toss gently.

CALORIES PER SERVING: 119   CARBS: 1 G
PROTEIN: 9 G   FAT: 8.75 G   SAT. FAT: 4 G

Snacks

Your snack choice should include protein and carbohydrates, for example, one stick of string cheese and one apple.

Late-Afternoon Snack Choices					
	Serving	Calories	Carbohydrates	Protein	Fat
Nonfat yogurt	6 oz	90	13.5	7.5	0
String cheese	1 oz	72	0	6	5
Beef jerky	2 oz	94	2	16	2
Turkey jerky	2 oz	90	2	16	0
Smoked fish	3 oz	80	0	19.5	0
Apple or pear	1	70	16	0	0
Protein bar (40-30-30 blend)	1	180	21	15	4
Peanuts or mixed nuts	1 oz	168	7	5	15

Dinner

Dinner may be the easiest meal to apply the three rules to. Most of you already have a type of cooking you enjoy. You can apply *No White at Night* to any style you enjoy, whether it is Asian, Italian, or Fusion. You simply need to remove the starch or starchy vegetables from your favorite recipes.

In the Gavin household, my mother often hosts a large dinner for three generations of the family. Her simple approach is to make dinner a lean protein such as meat, fish, or fowl, with two types of vegetables and a big salad. If you do not like salad, eat two vegetables. If you do not enjoy vegetables, consider making a huge salad. Remember, this is about foods that you like. When you choose your protein for your dinner meal, try to favor lean red meat, fish, or fowl. Try to avoid ground meat products, which could include a significant fat content. Fish that have dark flesh, such as salmon, steelhead, and tuna, are high in oils, especially omega-3 fatty acids that are favorable for lowering your risk of heart disease. Try to use cooking techniques that promote draining away any excess fat. Favor broiling or outdoor grilling, or use a George Foreman grill in the house.

Finally, remember that the *No White at Night* rule does not apply forever. After you have been able to achieve your target weight, you can reintroduce a portion of starch at your evening meal. That portion should be about the size of the palm of your hand. Try to favor starches that have a low glycemic index, although most will be similar in their glycemic load. Try to favor brown rice, sweet potatoes, or whole-wheat pastas. Most important, though, remember the concept of portion control.

Once you adopt these principles, you will find that your energy level and sense of well-being improve. You will no longer consider yourself "on a diet." You are likely, however, to change the way you eat for a lifetime.

Dinner Choices	
Lean protein	3–6 oz Meat/fish/fowl; serving size comparable to a chicken breast or a small steak
Nonstarchy vegetables	Unlimited
Salad	Unlimited; try to favor low-fat or nonfat salad dressing

No White at Night

Starches and high-starch vegetables to avoid at night include the following:

Bread of any type

Beans—lima, navy, pinto, red, refried

Corn

Pasta

Peas

Potatoes—red, sweet, white

Rice—brown or white

Squash—acorn, butternut

Bill's Favorite Braised Short Ribs

SERVES 6

3 lbs beef short ribs
salt and pepper to taste
2 Tbsp olive oil
1 large onion, finely chopped
1 carrot, finely chopped
1 stalk celery, finely chopped
12 cloves garlic, whole, peeled
1 Tbsp herbes de Provence
2 Tbsp flour
2 cups red wine, Merlot or Zinfandel
2½ cups beef broth
1 14-oz can diced tomatoes, either plain or with garlic and
   oregano
1 bay leaf
24 baby carrots, peeled
18 baby pearl onions, peeled
½ cup pitted and chopped Kalamata olives
salt and pepper to taste
3 Tbsp chopped fresh parsley, for garnish

✳ Preheat oven to 325 degrees. Sprinkle the beef ribs with salt and pepper to taste. In a heavy ovenproof pan, heat olive oil and brown the beef ribs. Put ribs aside, reserving 2 Tbsp of pan drippings, or add oil as necessary to make 2 Tbsp. Add onion, carrot, and celery and cook over medium-low heat until vegetables are soft, stirring frequently, about 10 minutes. Add garlic, herbes de Provence, and flour; stir 1 minute. Add wine and 2 cups broth; bring to a boil over high heat, scraping up browned bits. Add tomatoes with juices and bay leaf. Return ribs and any accumulated juices to pot. If necessary, add enough water to pot to barely cover the ribs. Bring to a boil.

Cover pot tightly and transfer to oven. Bake until ribs are very tender, stirring occasionally, about 2 hours 15 minutes. (Can be made one day ahead. Cool slightly, then refrigerate uncovered until cold. Cover and keep refrigerated. Take off fat. Bring to a simmer before continuing.)

Add pearl onions, carrots, olives, and remaining broth to pot; press carrots and onions gently to submerge. Cover, return to oven, and continue cooking at 350 degrees until carrots are tender, about 15 minutes. Discard bay leaf. Transfer short ribs and carrots to platter. Tent with foil to keep warm. If necessary, boil sauce to thicken slightly. Season to taste with salt and pepper. Pour sauce over short ribs. Garnish with parsley. Serve with Fauxtatoes Deluxe (page 135).

CALORIES PER SERVING: 362   CARBS: 21 G
PROTEIN: 52 G   FAT: 20 G   SAT. FAT: 10 G

Fauxtatoes Deluxe

1 large head cauliflower, or 2 16-oz bags frozen cauliflower
¼ cup reduced-fat cream or nonfat milk
4 oz nonfat cream cheese
1 Tbsp butter
salt and pepper to taste

✳ Simmer the cauliflower in water with the cream or milk added to it. (This keeps the cauliflower sweet and prevents it from turning an unappetizing gray color.) When the cauliflower is very soft, drain. Put the still-warm cauliflower in a food processor or blender with the cream cheese, butter, and salt and pepper to taste. Process until smooth. Alternately, for best results, mash by hand.

✳ For a lighter version, use 4–6 oz chicken broth instead of the cream and cream cheese.

CALORIES PER SERVING: 46   CARBS: 6 G
PROTEIN: 4 G   FAT: 10 G   SAT. FAT: 7 G

St. Raphael's Zesty Lime Chicken

⅓ cup fresh lime juice
2 tsp coarsely grated lime peel
¼ cup olive oil
2 Tbsp chopped pimento
2 cloves garlic, minced
1 ½ shakes hot sauce
⅓ cup chopped fresh cilantro
1 ½ tsp dried oregano
¾ tsp salt
¼ tsp black pepper
6 chicken breast halves, skinned and boned
lime slices and cilantro sprigs for garnish

✳ In large shallow glass baking dish, mix together lime juice, lime peel, olive oil, pimento, garlic, hot sauce, cilantro, oregano, salt, and pepper. Add chicken, turning to coat. Cover, place in the refrigerator, and marinate 30 minutes. Remove chicken from marinade and drain. Place marinade in a small saucepan and bring to a rolling boil. Place chicken in broiling pan. Set temperature control to broil. Arrange oven rack so chicken is about 7 inches from heat. Broil 20 minutes, turning once and brushing often with marinade. Brush chicken with marinade and broil additional 5 minutes or until a fork can be inserted in chicken with ease. Remove from broiler pan to serving dish and pour pan drippings over chicken. Garnish with lime slices and cilantro sprigs.

CALORIES PER SERVING: 166   CARBS: 6 G
PROTEIN: 22 G   FAT: 7.6 G   SAT. FAT: 0 G

Roger's Italian Clams

5–6 cloves garlic
1 Tbsp olive oil
1 ½ qt fresh manila clams, washed
1 tsp basil leaves

✳ Smash the garlic cloves with the side of a large carving knife (until the peel breaks) and place in olive oil in a large cast-iron or enamel skillet. Heat the skillet until it is very hot, the garlic turns brown, and the oil is about to smoke. Dump the clams in all at once. It will sound like popcorn popping. Cover and leave the heat up for about 3–5 minutes or until the clam shells have started to pop open. Lift the lid once and push the clams around a little bit. Cover for a few more minutes until most of the shells have opened. Lift the lid and sprinkle with the basil leaves. Continue to cook a few minutes more until the clams are done. (They will lose their shiny appearance.)

CALORIES PER SERVING: 217   CARBS: 2 G
PROTEIN: 12 G   FAT: 14 G   SAT. FAT: 2 G

Pakistan Chicken

½ cup plain nonfat yogurt
3 Tbsp minced onion
½ tsp minced garlic
½ tsp salt
¼ tsp crumbled, dried hot chili pepper
¼ tsp cumin
¼ tsp powdered ginger
⅛ tsp ground cardamom
⅛ tsp cinnamon
⅛ tsp powdered cloves
⅛ tsp black pepper
2 whole chicken breasts, skinned and boned
4 cherry tomatoes
1 red or yellow pepper, sliced

✳ Mix all ingredients, except tomatoes, peppers, and chicken, to make marinade. Cut chicken into pieces and marinate at least 4 hours. After marinating, put chicken on bamboo skewers with the tomatoes and peppers. Broil or grill until cooked through.

CALORIES PER SERVING: 287   CARBS: 8 G
PROTEIN: 64 G   FAT: 0 G   SAT. FAT: 0 G

Sesame Shrimp and Asparagus

1 ½ lb fresh asparagus
1 Tbsp sesame seeds
2 Tbsp olive oil
2 small onions, sliced
1 ½ lb shrimp, peeled, rinsed, and deveined
4 tsp soy sauce
1 ¼ tsp salt

✳ Break off ends of asparagus stalks, cut into 2-inch pieces, and set aside. In a 12-inch skillet over medium heat, toast sesame seeds; remove from pan. In same skillet over medium heat, add oil and cook asparagus, onion, and shrimp until shrimp are pink and vegetables are tender, about 5 minutes. Stir in sesame seeds, soy sauce, and salt.

CALORIES PER SERVING: 171   CARBS: 3 G
PROTEIN: 25 G   FAT: 6.5 G   SAT. FAT: 0 G

Jacki's Asparagus and Artichoke Soup

SERVES 10

4 medium onions, chopped

3 Tbsp butter

6 cups low-salt chicken broth

3 lb fresh asparagus, tough ends removed, tips removed and
reserved, chopped

2 14-oz cans artichoke bottoms or water-packed artichoke hearts,
chopped

light sour cream and chopped chives for garnish

✳ In large soup pot, sauté the onions in butter over medium heat until tender, about 10 minutes. Add the chicken broth, chopped asparagus, and chopped artichokes. Bring to a boil. Reduce heat and cook until tender. Purée the soup in batches in a food processor. Return to pot and heat. Ladle into bowls and top with a drizzle of the light sour cream and chives.

CALORIES PER SERVING: 113   CARBS: 16 G
PROTEIN: 4 G   FAT: 4 G   SAT. FAT: 2 G

Grilled Marinated Scallops

Juice of 8–10 limes or lemons
2 lb scallops
¼ cup olive oil
2 cloves garlic, minced
¼ cup finely chopped canned green chilies
¼ cup chopped fresh parsley
1 ½ tsp salt
1–2 dashes Tabasco sauce

✳ Up to 1 hour before cooking, pour lime juice over scallops in a large bowl to cover completely; add all the other ingredients and let stand in refrigerator 30–60 minutes. Do not marinate longer because the lime juice tends to cook the scallops. When ready to cook, drain the scallops and grill over a hot fire just until browned, 1–2 minutes. Serve.

CALORIES PER SERVING: 315   CARBS: 1.5 G
PROTEIN: 39 G   FAT: 17 G   SAT. FAT: 0 G

Korean BBQ Beef

¾ cup soy sauce
4 cloves garlic, minced
dash black pepper
2 green onions, finely chopped
2 Tbsp cooking oil
1 heaping Tbsp crushed sesame seeds
¼ cup sugar
3 lb rib steak of sirloin

✳ Combine all ingredients except the meat. Cut the meat into 1½-in cubes. Pour this mixture over the meat and work it into the meat. Marinate at least 1 hour. Cut the meat into chunks, put on bamboo skewers, and grill until done.

CALORIES PER SERVING: 288   CARBS: 1 G
PROTEIN: 32 G   FAT: 18 G   SAT. FAT: 9 G

Linnea's Tamari Teriyaki Marinade

¼ cup tamari soy sauce
1 ½ tsp honey
1 tsp minced fresh garlic
¼ tsp minced fresh ginger
2 Tbsp dry sherry
1 Tbsp minced onion

✳ Combine all ingredients in a small pan and bring to a simmer; remove from heat immediately and cool. Strain and use as a marinade for poultry and fish. Halibut is great.

CALORIES PER 1-TBSP SERVING: 62   CARBS: 15.5 G
PROTEIN: 0 G   FAT: 0 G   SAT. FAT: 0 G

Brennan's Flank Steak Marinade

2 cloves garlic, minced
¼ cup cooking oil
3 Tbsp soy sauce
2 Tbsp ketchup
1 Tbsp vinegar
¼ tsp black pepper

✳ Combine all ingredients. Marinate flank steak at least 3 hours or overnight. Broil about 6 inches from heat until browned; turn and brown other side.

CALORIES: 375   CARBS: 14 G
PROTEIN: 0 G   FAT: 42 G   SAT. FAT: 15 G

Chicken BBQ Marinade

¼ cup cooking oil
⅓ cup vinegar
⅔ cup orange juice
2 Tbsp Worcestershire sauce
⅓ cup ketchup
¼ cup minced onion
dash Tabasco sauce
2½ tsp salt
½ tsp chili powder
¼ tsp oregano

✳ Combine all ingredients. Marinate chicken at least 3 hours or overnight.

CALORIES PER 1-TBSP SERVING: 79   CARBS: 28 G
PROTEIN: 0 G   FAT: 7.5 G   SAT. FAT: 0 G

Yogurt Garlic Shrimp

½ Tbsp vegetable oil

8 cloves garlic, minced

¾ cup water

2 tsp cumin

1 tsp ground coriander

½ tsp turmeric

1 ½ lb large shrimp, peeled, rinsed, and deveined

2 tsp all-purpose flour

2 tsp sugar

½ tsp salt

1 8-oz carton plain nonfat yogurt

¼ cup green onion, sliced into 1-in pieces

✳ Heat oil in a large nonstick skillet over medium-high heat. Add garlic and cook until golden (about 30 seconds), stirring constantly. Stir in the water, cumin, coriander, and turmeric. Cover, reduce heat, and simmer 7 minutes. Add shrimp and cook 3 minutes. Combine flour, sugar, salt, and yogurt, and stir with a whisk. Stir yogurt mixture into the shrimp mixture. Cover and cook 4 minutes until shrimp are done. Stir in onions.

CALORIES PER SERVING: 245　CARBS: 12.7 G
PROTEIN: 30.3 G　FAT: 7.8 G　SAT. FAT: 1.4 G

Lemon Dill Flounder or Grouper

> 3 Tbsp butter
> 1 Tbsp chopped fresh dill
> 2 Tbsp fresh lemon juice
> ¼ tsp seasoned salt
> ¼ tsp white pepper
> 2 green onions, chopped
> 1 lb fresh flounder or grouper fillets

✳ Melt butter in a 10-inch skillet over medium heat. Add dill, lemon juice, salt, pepper, and onions. Sauté 5 minutes, stirring occasionally. Add fish and cook until firm but flaky, basting occasionally with pan juices, about 10–15 minutes.

CALORIES PER SERVING: 200   CARBS: 2 G
PROTEIN: 27 G   FAT: 9 G   SAT. FAT: 5 G

Mary's Carrot Salad

SERVES 4

1 clove garlic, minced
¼ tsp salt
¼ tsp black pepper, or to taste
1 Tbsp lemon juice
2 Tbsp olive oil
2 Tbsp chopped fresh parsley
3 large carrots, shredded

✳ Combine garlic, salt, pepper, lemon juice, olive oil, and parsley. Add the carrots and mix well.

> CALORIES PER SERVING: 85   CARBS: 4 G
> PROTEIN: 1.5 G   FAT: 7 G   SAT. FAT: 0 G

Spring Vegetable Mix

1 ½ cups cider vinegar

½ cup water

1 Tbsp sugar or sweetener

1 tsp salt, or to taste

1 tsp black peppercorns

½ tsp mustard seeds

½ tsp dried dill

2 bay leaves

2 cups small cauliflower florets

2 cups diagonally cut asparagus

1 ½ cups trimmed green beans

1 cup sliced carrots

1 cup sliced strips red bell pepper

6 green onions, sliced into 1 ½-in pieces

4 cloves garlic, peeled and halved

✳ Combine vinegar, water, sugar, salt, peppercorns, mustard seeds, dill, and bay leaves in a large pan. Bring to a boil, reduce heat, and simmer 3 minutes. Arrange remaining ingredients in a large heavy-duty zip-top plastic bag. Carefully pour vinegar mixture over cauliflower mixture. Seal bag and refrigerate 8 hours or overnight, turning occasionally. Remove vegetables from bag with a slotted spoon. Discard bay leaves.

CALORIES PER SERVING: 57 CARBS: 13 G
PROTEIN: 3.2 G FAT: 3 G SAT. FAT: 0 G

Liz's Stuffed Green Peppers

> *2 Tbsp olive oil*
> *1 large eggplant, peeled and cut into ½-in cubes*
> *1 ½ cups tomato sauce*
> *8 Tbsp grated Parmesan cheese*
> *2 cloves garlic, crushed*
> *2 large green peppers, seeded and cut in half*

✳ Preheat oven to 350 degrees. Heat olive oil in a pan and fry eggplant until soft. Mix with the tomato sauce, 4 Tbsp cheese, and garlic. Cook the peppers in salted boiling water for 5 minutes. Drain and fill with the eggplant mixture. Sprinkle with the remaining cheese. Bake 20 minutes.

CALORIES PER SERVING: 138   CARBS: 11 G
PROTEIN: 2 G   FAT: 12 G   SAT. FAT: 2.5 G

Betsy's Green Beans

SERVES 4

1 lb fresh green beans
3 Tbsp olive oil
4 cloves garlic, minced
½ tsp dried chilies
1 ½ tsp sugar
½ tsp salt
½ tsp whole black mustard seed (optional)

✳ Parboil beans, cool in cold water, strain, and set aside. Heat olive oil in a pan and add garlic, chilies, sugar, salt, and mustard seed, if desired. Add the green beans. Mix and stir-fry 8–10 minutes. Serve warm or cold.

CALORIES PER SERVING: 118   CARBS: 5 G
PROTEIN: 1 G   FAT: 10 G   SAT. FAT: 0 G

Oriental Vegetable Stir-Fry

1 Tbsp rice vinegar

1 Tbsp low-sodium soy sauce

1 tsp curry powder

½ tsp salt

⅛ tsp black pepper

2 Tbsp tomato paste

1 ½ Tbsp vegetable oil

1 sweet onion, cut into 8 wedges

1 cup chopped celery

½ cup water

¼ cup sliced water chestnuts, drained

1 medium zucchini, quartered lengthwise and sliced thick

1 medium yellow squash, quartered lengthwise and sliced thick

2 cups ¼-in-thick sliced green or red peppers

2 cups thinly sliced Napa cabbage

1 Tbsp slivered almonds

❋ Combine rice vinegar, soy sauce, curry powder, salt, pepper, and tomato paste in a small bowl; set aside. Heat oil in a stir-fry pan or wok over medium heat. Add onion and celery and stir-fry 1 minute. Increase heat to medium-high, add water and water chestnuts, zucchini, yellow squash, and peppers and stir-fry 3 minutes. Add tomato paste mixture; bring to boil and cook 1 minute. Stir in cabbage and almonds.

CALORIES PER SERVING: 102   CARBS: 10.8 G
PROTEIN: 2.5 G   FAT: 6.5 G   SAT. FAT: 1.1 G

Cioppino

1 ½ lb red snapper or halibut
½ Tbsp olive oil
1 ½ cups chopped onion
3–4 cloves garlic, minced
1 cup thinly sliced mushrooms
1 cup coarsely chopped green pepper
4 cups chopped tomatoes
¼ cup dry red wine
¼ cup clam juice
2 bay leaves
¾ tsp dried basil
¼ tsp freshly ground black pepper
2 Tbsp chopped fresh parsley
3–4 dashes hot sauce
½ lb medium shrimp, peeled, rinsed, and deveined
½ tsp salt
juice of 1 lemon

✳ Cut fish into 2-inch cubes and set aside. In a heavy stock-pot, heat olive oil and add onion, garlic, mushrooms, and green pepper. Sauté about 5 minutes. Add tomatoes, wine, clam juice, bay leaves, basil, black pepper, parsley, and hot sauce. Simmer 15 minutes. Add fish and cook gently 25 minutes, stirring occasionally. Add shrimp and cook 8 minutes, stirring occasionally. Season with salt and lemon juice. Serve in warmed soup bowls.

CALORIES PER SERVING: 109   CARBS: 5 G
PROTEIN: 17 G   FAT: 2 G   SAT. FAT: 0 G

Roasted Carrot & Onion Soup

SERVES 2

1 Tbsp olive oil
12 oz carrots, peeled and cut into ½-in rounds
1 large onion, chopped
2 cloves garlic, chopped
¼ tsp dried thyme
3 cups canned low-salt chicken broth
salt and pepper to taste
fresh chives, minced, or green onion tops, chopped, for garnish

✳ Preheat over to 375 degrees. Heat olive oil in an ovenproof skillet. Add carrots and onion and sauté until onion is tender, about 10 minutes. Transfer to the oven and bake until vegetables start to brown, about 45 minutes, stirring occasionally. Remove skillet from oven and add garlic, thyme, and broth. Cover and simmer until the carrots are very tender, about 30 minutes. Transfer to blender and purée until smooth. Add more broth if mixture is too thick. Bring soup to a simmer and season with salt and pepper to taste. Ladle into bowls and garnish with chives or green onions.

This soup can be made up to two days ahead.

CALORIES PER SERVING: 128 CARBS: 13.5 G
PROTEIN: 9 G FAT: 9.5 G SAT. FAT: 0 G

Caramelized Onion Soup

8 cups thinly sliced white onions
1 Tbsp olive oil
⅓ cup butter
1 ¼ lb thinly sliced mushrooms
½ cup white wine
½ cup brandy
6 cups chicken or vegetable stock
½ tsp fresh thyme
¼ tsp Italian parsley, chopped
salt and black pepper to taste
Parmesan cheese, grated, for garnish
parsley, chopped, for garnish

❋ Slowly cook the onions in olive oil until caramelized. Add butter and mushrooms and cook until the mushrooms are done. In a separate pan, mix wine and brandy and reduce by one-third. Add to the onions. Add stock and bring to a boil, then reduce to a simmer. Add thyme, Italian parsley, and salt and pepper to taste. Simmer 30 minutes and add more herbs, salt and pepper to taste. Ladle into bowls and garnish with Parmesan cheese and parsley.

CALORIES PER SERVING: 201   CARBS: 27 G
PROTEIN: 2.4 G   FAT: 9 G   SAT. FAT: 0 G

Marinated Vegetable Salad

2 red peppers, cut in half

2 yellow crookneck squash, sliced thin lengthwise

2 zucchini, sliced thin lengthwise

2 Japanese eggplants, sliced thin lengthwise

olive oil

2 Tbsp chopped fresh basil

1 tsp oregano

1 tsp parsley

1 tsp thyme

3 cloves garlic, pressed

salt and black pepper

1 Tbsp olive oil

1 ½ Tbsp balsamic vinegar

3 tomatoes, sliced thin

2 Tbsp chopped Kalamata olives

✳ Preheat broiler. Arrange the peppers, cut side down. Broil until skin blackens. Transfer the peppers to a bag and cool. When cool, peel the peppers and slice thin. Arrange the squash, zucchini, and eggplant on a baking sheet and brush with olive oil. Broil about 4 minutes per side. Mix all the herbs in a small bowl along with the garlic. Layer the vegetables, seasoning with salt and pepper and drizzling with oil, vinegar, and the herb mixture for each layer. Save one-fifth of the herb mixture for later. Cover the vegetables and chill overnight. Let stand 1 hour at room temperature. For the last layer arrange tomato slices atop the vegetables. Season with salt and pepper and drizzle with oil, vinegar, and the last of the herb mix. Top with the olives.

CALORIES PER SERVING: 235   CARBS: 35 G
PROTEIN: 4.25 G   FAT: 21.4 G   SAT. FAT: 0 G

Dominic's Herb-Crusted Pork Tenderloin with Fruit Salsa

SERVES 4

12–14 large strawberries, minced

1 papaya, minced

1 red onion, minced

½ cup chopped fresh cilantro

1 ½ Tbsp lime juice

1 tsp salt

1 tsp marjoram

1 tsp oregano

1 tsp basil

1 tsp thyme

2 Tbsp olive oil

1 12-oz pork tenderloin or loin roast

❋ Combine the strawberries, papaya, onion, cilantro, lime juice, and salt in a glass bowl and refrigerate overnight to blend the flavors. Preheat oven to 375 degrees. Mix herbs in a small bowl. Pour the olive oil into a glass baking dish, roll the pork in it to cover with oil, and rub with the herb mixture. Bake the pork 40–45 minutes or until the inner temperature is 160 degrees. Slice the pork into ¼- to ½-in slices and serve with the strawberry salsa, warmed to room temperature.

CALORIES PER SERVING: 292 CARBS: 17 G
PROTEIN: 25.5 G   FAT: 11 G   SAT. FAT: 3 G

Roasted Fennel, Tomato, and Chicken Casserole

SERVES 2

2 chicken breasts, skinned, boned, and chopped
2 Tbsp extra-virgin olive oil
2 medium fennel bulbs, washed and trimmed
1 head garlic, cloves peeled and, if large, halved
1 Tbsp chopped fennel seeds
4 canned plum tomatoes, chopped (about ⅔ cup)
¼ tsp dried chili flakes
salt and freshly ground black pepper to taste
1 cup loosely packed basil leaves
½ cup cubed fresh mozzarella cheese (about 3 oz)
⅓ cup freshly grated Parmesan cheese

✳ Preheat oven to 450 degrees. Brown the chicken in 1 Tbsp olive oil; set aside. Cut the fennel bulbs into quarters through their cores. With a chef's knife, cut out each core, set the wedges cut side down, and cut them into ⅛-in slices. In a shallow ovenproof dish, toss the fennel with the garlic, fennel seeds, the remaining olive oil, tomatoes, chili flakes, and salt and pepper to taste. Spread the mixture evenly in the bottom of the pan and add the chicken. Roast without stirring until the fennel is limp and somewhat browned, 35–45 minutes. Tear the basil leaves into pieces and add them to the pot. Just before serving, toss with the mozzarella and Parmesan cheese.

CALORIES PER SERVING: 303   CARBS: 5 G
PROTEIN: 30 G   FAT: 18 G   SAT FAT: 6 G

Portobello Mushroom Caps

SERVES 2

2 4-in portobello mushrooms
2 Tbsp chopped sun-dried tomatoes
2 Tbsp chopped Kalamata olives
2 tsp chopped fresh basil
2 tsp chopped garlic
½ cup grated mozzarella cheese

✳ Wipe mushrooms clean and place belly side up on foil-lined broiler. Sprinkle with tomatoes, olives, basil, and garlic. Top with cheese and broil until cooked through, approximately 15 minutes.

CALORIES PER SERVING: 175   CARBS: 5.5 G
PROTEIN: 17 G   FAT: 9.5 G   SAT. FAT: 0 G

Auntie Laur's Seared Scallops over Spinach (Father Pollard's Favorite)

2 Tbsp canola oil

2 tsp toasted sesame oil

2 cloves garlic, minced

1 1-in piece ginger, minced or grated

1 6-oz bag spinach

1 Tbsp soy sauce

1 ½ Tbsp toasted sesame seeds

freshly ground black pepper to taste

1 ½ lbs scallops

✴ Heat 1 Tbsp canola oil and 1 tsp sesame oil in a skillet over high heat. Add garlic and ginger and cook until soft, about 1 minute. Add spinach and cook until tender, about 2 minutes. Add soy sauce, sesame seeds, and pepper. Toss to combine. Keep warm. Heat the remaining canola oil and sesame oil over medium-high heat in a skillet. Sear scallops until golden (about 2 minutes per side). Serve over spinach.

CALORIES PER SERVING: 227 G   CARBS: 2.5 G
PROTEIN: 23 G   FAT: 11 G   SAT. FAT: 0 G

Carolyn's Famous Tonnato Sauce

1 6-oz can water-packed albacore tuna, drained
2 Tbsp nonfat plain yogurt
juice of ½ lemon
2 Tbsp light olive oil
1 tsp minced garlic
fresh parsley to taste
freshly ground black pepper to taste
capers (optional)

✴ Combine all ingredients in a food processor and process until mixture is well blended and creamy. Add more yogurt and olive oil if a smoother texture is preferred. Use on veal, chicken, or turkey, or as a vegetable dip.

CALORIES PER 1-TBSP SERVING: 106   CARBS: 1 G
PROTEIN: 9 G   FAT: 30 G   SAT. FAT: 4 G

Grilled Tuna

1 ½ cups chopped and seeded tomatoes (about 1 ½ lb)
¾ cup chopped fresh parsley
¼ cup chopped and pitted Niçoise olives
1 Tbsp white wine vinegar
¼ tsp dried tarragon
¼ tsp salt
2 cloves garlic, minced
4 6-oz tuna steaks
1 ½ tsp herbes de Provence
¼ tsp salt
cooking spray
chive sprigs for garnish (optional)

✳ Combine tomatoes, parsley, olives, vinegar, tarragon, salt, and garlic in a medium bowl. Cover and chill 20 minutes. Prepare grill. Sprinkle the fish with herbes de Provence and salt. Place fish on a grill rack coated with cooking spray; cook 3 minutes on each side or until fish is medium-rare or to desired degree of doneness. Serve fish with tomato mixture. Garnish with chive sprigs, if desired.

CALORIES PER SERVING: 278   CARBS: 5 G
PROTEIN: 40.8 G   FAT: 9.7 G   SAT. FAT: 2.4 G

Florida Citrus Grilled Tuna

1 lemon
1 lime
1 cup water
1 Tbsp rice wine vinegar
2 Tbsp sliced shallots
2 cloves garlic, minced
1 ½ tsp sugar
1 Tbsp olive oil
¼ tsp crushed red pepper
2 tuna steaks (at least 1-in thick and about 8 oz)
olive oil or cooking spray
cilantro sprigs for garnish

✳ For vinaigrette: Peel the zest from the lemon and the lime. Julienne the zest. Bring a cup of water to boil and drop the zest in for 30 seconds. Rinse with cold water and drain. Juice the lemon and lime and combine the juice with the zest, vinegar, shallots, garlic, sugar, oil, and red pepper. Coat the tuna steaks lightly with oil or cooking spray. Grill 2–3 minutes per side, basting with a little vinaigrette. Serve with remaining vinaigrette. Garnish with cilantro sprigs.

CALORIES PER SERVING: 327   CARBS: 4 G
PROTEIN: 50 G   FAT: 4 G   SAT. FAT: 0.5 G

Mom's Coleslaw

4 cups thinly sliced cabbage
3 Tbsp nonfat or low-fat mayonnaise
3 Tbsp rice, cider, or white vinegar
1 tsp sugar or sweetener
dash Tabasco sauce
black pepper to taste
½ tsp poultry seasoning
shredded carrot or green pepper (optional)

✳ Combine all ingredients and toss.

CALORIES PER SERVING: 186   CARBS: 46.5 G
PROTEIN: 6 G   FAT: 2 G   SAT. FAT: O G

Chicken Lettuce Wraps

SERVES 4

2 chicken breast halves, skinned and boned
2 tsp olive oil
2 Tbsp grated fresh ginger
2 Tbsp soy sauce
1 Tbsp honey
2 Tbsp rice vinegar
½ tsp crushed red pepper
½ tsp cornstarch
1 cup fresh bean sprouts
1 ½ cups grated carrot
1 cup snow peas, sliced into strips
½ cup slivered bamboo shoots
½ cup chopped green onion
¼ cup toasted slivered almonds
12 Bibb lettuce leaves
1 Tbsp toasted sesame seeds

✳ Chop chicken into small chunks. Heat oil in a skillet over medium-high heat. Sauté chicken 5 minutes or until chicken is done. Combine soy sauce, honey, vinegar, red pepper, ginger, and cornstarch and whisk together. Add to chicken. Then stir in bean sprouts, carrot, snow peas, bamboo shoots, and onion. Cook about 3 minutes or until the sauce thickens, stirring often. Add almonds. Spoon ¼ cup of the mixture onto each of the lettuce leaves, sprinkle with sesame seeds, and serve with any Asian dipping or peanut sauce.

CALORIES PER SERVING: 267   CARBS: 17 G
PROTEIN: 22 G   FAT: 12.1 G   SAT. FAT: 0 G

Peanut Marinade or Sauce

MAKES 1 CUP

½ cup chunky peanut butter
½ cup peanut oil
¼ cup white wine vinegar
¼ cup tamari or soy sauce
¼ cup lemon juice
1 clove garlic, minced
8 sprigs cilantro, minced
2 tsp dried red pepper flakes
2 tsp chopped fresh ginger

❋ Combine all ingredients in a blender and process until smooth, adding a few drops of water if mixture is too thick. May reserve one half of the marinade. Do this prior to adding the meat since it is not wise to reuse marinade after raw meat has been added. Marinate beef or chicken overnight. Grill. Serve marinade as a dipping sauce if desired.

CALORIES PER 1-TBSP SERVING: 75   CARBS: 1 G
PROTEIN: 1.5 G   FAT: 7.7 G   SAT. FAT: 1.5 G

Cottage Cheese Dressing

MAKES 1½ CUPS

1 cup low-fat cottage cheese
⅓ cup low-fat buttermilk

❋ Process in blender or Cuisinart until smooth.
For dill dressing, add ½–1 tsp dried dill weed.
For blue cheese dressing, add 1 Tbsp blue cheese and black pepper to taste.
For green goddess dressing, add 3 anchovies, 1 tsp chopped green onion, 1 Tbsp chopped fresh parsley, and chopped tarragon to taste.

CALORIES: 12 CARBS: 1 G

PROTEIN: 2 G FAT: 0 G SAT. FAT: 0 G

Vinaigrette

❋ To make a simple low-fat dressing, blend extra-virgin olive oil with balsamic vinegar, Italian herbs, and minced garlic. This can be changed to a citrus vinaigrette by using rice vinegar and orange or lemon juice with a sweetener.

CALORIES PER 1-TBSP SERVING: 130 CARBS: 0 G

PROTEIN: 0 G FAT: 14 G SAT. FAT: 0 G

Mary's Vinaigrette

1 ½ cups olive oil
½ cup balsamic or red wine vinegar
2 tsp salt
1 tsp freshly ground black pepper
1 tsp sugar
1 Tbsp grated onion
1 clove garlic, minced

✳ Combine all ingredients and shake well.

CALORIES PER 2-TBSP SERVING: 94   CARBS: 1 G
PROTEIN: 0 G   FAT: 10 G   SAT. FAT: 0 G

Tofu Spread

1 Tbsp Dijon mustard
½ Tbsp cider vinegar
1 Tbsp minced onion
¼ cup water
10 oz tofu
freshly ground black pepper to taste

✳ Combine all ingredients in a food processor and process until smooth.

CALORIES PER 2-TBSP SERVING: 13.7
CARBS: 1 G   PROTEIN: 1 G   FAT: 0.5 G   SAT. FAT: 0 G

Cold Lemon Asparagus

2 cloves garlic, minced
2 tsp Dijon mustard
3 Tbsp fresh lemon juice
2 Tbsp olive oil
½ tsp sugar
salt and pepper to taste
2 lb asparagus
2 Tbsp chopped fresh parsley
½ tsp sea salt (optional)

✳ Combine garlic, mustard, and lemon juice and whisk together. Slowly drizzle in the olive oil, stirring constantly. Add the sugar and salt and pepper to taste. Heat a large skillet with water, and sea salt if desired, over medium-high heat. Bring to a boil, add the asparagus in small batches, and cook until tender. As each batch cooks, rinse in cold water. When ready to serve, arrange asparagus on a plate, drizzle with vinaigrette, sprinkle with parsley, and serve.

CALORIES PER SERVING: 110   CARBS: 6 G
PROTEIN: 3.5 G   FAT: 4.5 G   SAT. FAT: 0.5 G

Andre's Pork Tenderloin with Brown Sauce

> 2 Tbsp olive oil
> 2 ½ lb pork tenderloin
> 1 tsp thyme and other herbs, chopped

✹ Preheat oven to 325 degrees. Add olive oil to a large skillet over high heat. Brown the pork on all sides. Place in a baking dish and sprinkle with herbs. Bake the pork 30 minutes or until the inner temperature is 170 degrees. Let the pork rest about 10 minutes. Slice the pork in ½-in slices and place on a plate with 2 Tbsp Brown Sauce.

Brown Sauce

> 1 oz butter
> 2 Tbsp finely chopped shallots
> 2–3 stalks celery, finely chopped
> 3–4 parsley sprigs, finely chopped
> 2 Tbsp flour
> 1 10½-oz can beef consommé
> ½ can water
> 3-oz can tomato paste
> 6 oz red wine
> salt and black pepper to taste

✹ Melt butter in a skillet and sauté shallots, celery, and parsley until softened. Add the flour and stir to blend. Add consommé, water, tomato paste, and wine, whisking to keep smooth. Add salt and pepper to taste. Bring to a boil, then reduce heat and cook about 15 minutes. Strain.

CALORIES PER SERVING: 245   CARBS: 5 G
PROTEIN: 21 G   FAT: 15.6 G   SAT. FAT: 7 G

Grilled Vegetables Marinade

MAKES ¾ CUP

¼ cup olive oil
¼ cup balsamic vinegar
4 cloves garlic, minced
¼ cup water
salt and pepper to taste
assorted vegetables cut for grilling: onions, zucchini, asparagus,
    eggplant, peppers, portobello mushrooms

✳ Combine oil, vinegar, garlic, water, and salt and pepper to taste. Whisk together. Drizzle the oil mixture over the vegetables at least 1 hour prior to grilling. People usually think of grilling meats. Vegetables are great on the grill, so the next time you are cooking a steak, try doing the vegetables as well.

CALORIES: 119   CARBS: 9 G
PROTEIN: 3 G   FAT: 13 G   SAT. FAT: 2 G

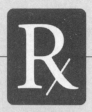

✳ *Exercise—walk one half hour per day*

✳ *Eat three meals per day*

✳ *Eat some lean protein with every meal*

✳ *No white at night*

Place this page on your refrigerator door.

NOTES

1. Sears, Barry, Ph.D. *The Zone Diet.* New York: Regan Books, 1995.
2. Centers for Disease Control. National Center for Health Statistics. *Overweight Prevalence Statistics,* 1999.
3. Fontaine, K. R., D. T. Redden, C. Wang, A. O. Westfall, and D. B. Allison. Years of life lost due to obesity. *JAMA* 289:187–193, 2003.
4. Serdula, M. K., A. H. Mokdad, D. F. Williamson, D. A. Galuska, J. M. Mendlein, and G. W. Heath. Prevalence of attempting weight loss and strategies for controlling weight. *JAMA* 282:1353–1358, 1999.

5. Maskalyk, J. Southern Africa's famine far worse than anticipated. *CMAJ* 167:11–12, 2002.

6. Cordain, L. *The Paleo Diet.* New York: Wiley, 2002.

7. Irwin, M. C., Y. Yasui, C. M. Ulrich, D. Bowen, et al. Effect of exercise on total and intra-abdominal body fat in postmenopausal women. *JAMA* 289: 323–330, 2003.

8. Atkins, R. C. *Dr. Atkins' New Diet Revolution.* New York: Avon Books, 1992.

9. Ludwig, D. S. The glycemic index. *JAMA* 287: 2414–2423, 2002.

10. Brand-Miller, J. *The New Glucose Revolution.* New York: Marlowe, 2003.

11. Mokdad, A. H., E. S. Ford, B. A. Bowman, et. al. Prevalence of obesity, diabetes, and obesity-related health risk factors, 2001. *JAMA* 289:76–79, 2003.